healthy eating for
lower blood pressure

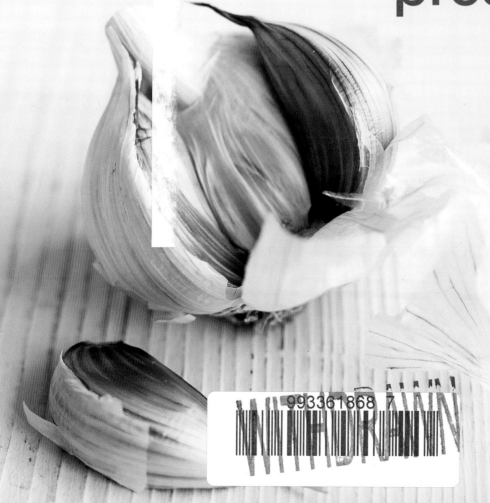

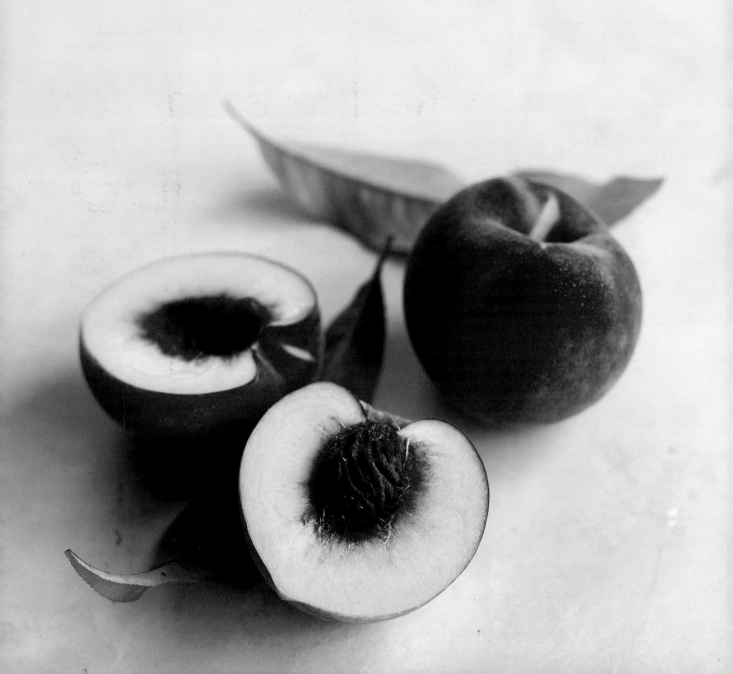

Paul Gayler with
Gemma Heiser

healthy eating for
lower blood
pressure

For the first time, a chef and a nutritionist have teamed up
to inspire you with over 100 delicious recipes

Photography by Will Heap

Kyle Cathie Ltd

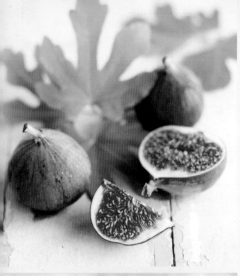

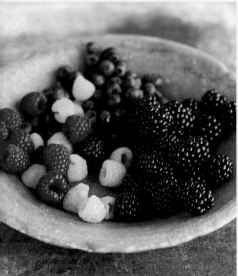

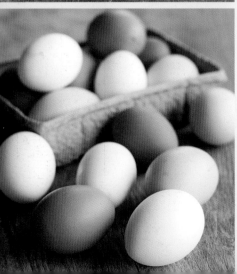

Dedication

To the many of you that suffer from high blood pressure but enjoy good food,
this book is for you.
Good health and good eating!!

First published in Great Britain in 2010 by
Kyle Cathie Limited
23 Howland Street, London W1T 4AY
general.enquiries@kyle-cathie.com
www.kylecathie.com

ISBN: 978-1-85626-922-3

A CIP catalogue record for this title is available from the British Library.

10 9 8 7 6 5 4 3 2 1

Project Editor: Judith Hannam
Design: geoffhayes@mac.com
Copy Editor: Debra Stottor
Proofreader: Gill Lange
Indexer: Peter Lange
Photographer: Will Heap
Home Economists: Linda Tubby
Prop Stylist: Roisin Nield
Production: Gemma John
Colour reproduction: SC (Sang Choy) Internatio
Printed and bound in Singapore by Star Standard Industries Pte Ltd

contents

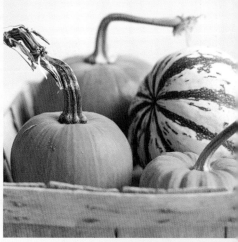

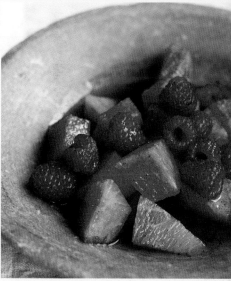

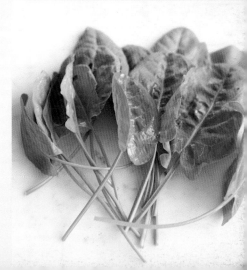

foreword

High blood pressure is one of the most pressing health problems of the modern day. In the UK it is estimated that around 15 million people have high blood pressure with almost 5 million of those being unaware of it. Awareness is the vital first step. The good news is that if you know you have high blood pressure or are at risk of high blood pressure there are things that you can do about it. If you have been diagnosed with high blood pressure and put onto medication by your doctor – take them. But also remember that the way you live your life also has a massive impact on your health. Poor diet and an excess of salt are a major cause of high blood pressure and changes in your diet can bring down your blood pressure quite dramatically.

This book can help you lower your blood pressure. By following the advice and recipes, it will help you to change your diet in a way which will help lower your blood pressure – and without foregoing any pleasure.

By re-educating your taste buds you will learn to live with a lot less salt. Adding extra portions of fruit and vegetables to your diet to meet or exceed the '5 a day' target will help you significantly reduce the risk of stroke and heart disease. Increasing the amount of potassium rich foods in your diet will have a direct impact on your blood pressure.

Using the knowledge collected in this book will help you reduce your blood pressure and as a result reduce your risk of stroke and heart disease. If you have been diagnosed with high blood pressure, this book will help you control it. Follow the advice and recipes closely and you will notice a difference.

Michael Rich
Blood Pressure Association

a chef's prescription

Are you one of those people who think that healthy food can't possibly taste good? Does the idea of eating healthily instil fear and conjure up all manner of images of dull, boring and uninspiring food, akin to rabbit food?

Sadly, healthy eating over the years has come to be associated with the vast amount of faddy diets that don't do you any good at all. To me, there is no such thing as a diet, only a lifestyle change.

As a chef I love to cook, and love to eat good food, and I see no reason why a healthy diet should not be an interesting one. Eating is one of life's greatest pleasures and eating healthy foods should be as much fun as eating not-so-healthy foods.

However, we often find it difficult to make changes in our lives and our eating habits are no exception. We know in our minds that we should and could be eating better but often it seems too much of a monumental upheaval and it's difficult to know where to start.

Eating healthily can benefit us all, but it is especially relevant for those with high blood pressure. What you eat can greatly affect your chances of developing high blood pressure and a healthy eating regime can both reduce the risk of developing it and lower a blood pressure that is already too high.

So what do we need to do to make healthy eating a reality?

It can be accomplished by simply changing our eating habits, varying the methods we use to cook and understanding how to get the maximum flavour from food. We need to be aware of the dangers of certain foods, especially those high in salt, saturated fat and added sugar, and save them for a special occasion. There's no need to cut out all your favourite foods completely, like always denying yourself French fries in favour of yet another healthy green salad leaf! It is just about getting the balance right.

The main thing is to explore the incredible variety of healthy ingredients that are available to us and that we should be eating more often. Many types of fresh fish, together with fruit and vegetables are all nutritious foods just waiting to give endless variation to the food we eat everyday and add tasty and exotic dishes to your repertoire. Start by integrating small changes to your eating habits, ones that are easy to achieve and stick to, and before you know it you will be eating healthier and feeling better in yourself.

Cut back on those foods that give you saturated fat, added sugars and calories but little else. Choose leaner cuts of meat, such as low-fat chicken, fish and an abundance of fruit and vegetables and reduce salt in your diet by cooking with alternative spices and flavourings for really knock-out, delicious food.

This book sets out to inform and inspire you to experience new foods while at the same time improving your health. There is certainly no need to cook bland and boring dishes with the many options available in the book.

And on a final note, all new things take a while to adapt to, so be patient and change your diet gradually if you find that easier. Follow a balanced diet, make informed and healthy choices with everything that that you eat, at all times, whether it be a quick snack or a planned meal.

And most importantly, be careful not to over-analyse your diet as this will take all the pleasure out of good eating. Eat sensibly and you'll feel better for it.

Good health, bon appetite!!

Paul….

introduction

High blood pressure is the biggest known cause of disability and premature death in the UK through stroke, heart attack and heart disease. One in three adults in the UK have high blood pressure and every day 350 people have a preventable stroke or heart attack caused by the condition. It also increases the risk of kidney and eye disease, dementia and other illnesses.

If your blood pressure is too high you may be very concerned about these risks. But the good news is there is a lot you can do to lower your blood pressure and keep it that way. Making some simple diet and lifestyle changes can have a real effect on your blood pressure and help you avoid these health problems in the future.

Even if you do not have high blood pressure, it is important to keep your blood pressure as low as you can. The lower your blood pressure the better for avoiding health problems in the future.

This book will show you how you can take control of your blood pressure and dramatically reduce your risk of a future stroke or heart attack.

about blood pressure

When your heart beats it pumps blood around your body to give it the energy and oxygen it needs. As the blood moves it pushes against the sides of your blood vessels. The strength of this pushing is your blood pressure.

If your blood pressure is too high it puts a strain on your body. Over many months and years this extra strain can cause damage to your heart and blood vessels which increases your risk of a stroke or heart attack.

When your blood pressure is measured it will be written as two numbers, for example 120/80mmHg. You would read this as '120 over 80' (mmHg stands for 'millimetres of mercury' which are the units used to measure blood pressure). The two numbers show the highest and lowest pressures in your blood vessels:

● The first (or top) number is your systolic blood pressure. This is the highest level your blood pressure reaches when your heart beats
● The second (or bottom) number is your diastolic blood pressure. This is the lowest level your blood pressure reaches between heart beats

Both of these numbers are very important – the higher they are, the higher your risk of health problems in the future.

WHAT DO MY BLOOD PRESSURE NUMBERS MEAN?
Look at figure 1 to see what your blood pressure numbers mean. Find your top number (systolic pressure) on the left side of the chart and read across. Find your bottom number (diastolic pressure) on the bottom of the chart and read up. Where the two meet is your blood pressure.

Table 1 gives more detailed information on your blood pressure readings and what to do about them.

Figure 1
WHAT SHOULD MY BLOOD PRESSURE BE?
You can see from table 1 health professionals agree that a healthy blood pressure is 120/80 or lower (but not below 90/60 which could mean you have low blood pressure). Lower blood pressure puts less strain on your heart and blood vessels which reduces your risk of health problems.

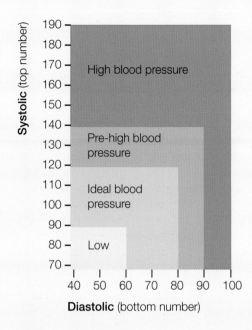

Systolic (top number) — Diastolic (bottom number)

- High blood pressure
- Pre-high blood pressure
- Ideal blood pressure
- Low

A person with a blood pressure of 115/75 has half the risk of having a stroke or heart attack as a person with a blood pressure of 135/85.

If your blood pressure is 140/90 or above you may have high blood pressure – visit your GP surgery for advice.

KNOW YOUR NUMBERS – GET CHECKED!
There are usually no symptoms of high blood pressure. Many people with high blood pressure do not know they have it – they have not thought to get a blood pressure check because they feel perfectly well. This is why it is so important for you to know your blood pressure numbers. Having a blood pressure check is simple, painless and allows you to take action before it is too late.

All adults should have their blood pressure checked at least every five years. If you have high blood pressure, or your readings are higher than they should be, you may need to have more frequent checks. Your doctor or nurse will advise you.

Table 1: What your blood pressure numbers mean

Your reading	What this means	What to do now
90/60 or below	You may have low blood pressure	Visit your GP surgery for advice
91/61 to 120/80	Your blood pressure is ideal	Follow diet and lifestyle advice in this book to help keep it at this ideal level
121/81 to 129/84	Your blood pressure is a little higher than it should be	Try to lower your blood pressure - follow the diet and lifestyle advice in this book
130/85 to 139/89	Your blood pressure is higher than it should be and could soon become high blood pressure	Try to lower your blood pressure as much as possible – follow the diet and lifestyle advice in this book
140/90 or above	You may have high blood pressure	Visit your GP surgery for advice. Follow the diet and lifestyle advice in this book

high blood pressure

Diagnosis

A single high reading of 140/90 or above does not mean you have high blood pressure. Many things affect your blood pressure so your doctor will take a number of readings at different times to see if it stays high. If your blood pressure is always 140/90 or more over time, your doctor will diagnose high blood pressure. Your doctor will also diagnose high blood pressure if only one of your readings is always higher than it should be. For example, if your blood pressure is 145/85 with only your top number (systolic pressure) being higher than it should be.

Causes

For a very small number of people with high blood pressure (around five per cent) there is an underlying health problem which, if treated, can lower their blood pressure back to normal. Your doctor will rule out any underlying problems with a few simple tests.

But for most people there is probably no single cause of their high blood pressure. What we do know is that certain lifestyle factors put you at risk of developing the condition including:

- Eating too much salt
- Not eating enough fruit and vegetables
- Being overweight
- Not being active enough
- Drinking too much alcohol

There are some other factors you cannot control which also increase your risk of developing high blood pressure. These include having a family history of high blood pressure, being from African-Caribbean or South Asian communities or getting older (the effects of an unhealthy lifestyle can build up over the years to put you at higher risk).

Treatment

For people with high blood pressure the aim is usually to get it down to 140/85 or below. But if you also have other health problems like kidney disease or diabetes, or you have had a stroke or heart attack, your doctor or nurse may advise you to aim for a lower target than this.

If you have high blood pressure, or your blood pressure is higher than ideal, making some diet and lifestyle changes could help you lower it back to healthy levels. But sometimes this is not enough. If this applies to you, you might also need to take medicines to help lower your blood pressure further. You might also need to take medicines if you have a higher risk of stroke and heart attack, for example if you smoke or have a family history of heart disease.

Even if you do need to take blood pressure medicines you can still benefit from making changes to your diet and lifestyle which could help your medicines work better and reduce your risk of future health problems.

For more information on living with high blood pressure, including measuring blood pressure, treatment options and blood pressure lowering ideas see the Blood Pressure Association's website: www.bpassoc.org.uk

Key points

- High blood pressure increases the risk of stroke and heart attack if left untreated
- Lowering blood pressure as much as possible helps reduce your risk of future health problems
- This means making diet and lifestyle changes and taking medicines if you need to

a healthy balanced diet

Eating a healthy balanced diet can benefit everyone but is especially important if you have high blood pressure. Making simple changes to your diet can lower your blood pressure and help reduce your risk of future health problems.

If your blood pressure is higher than it should be, making changes to what you eat could make all the difference between needing to take blood pressure medicines or not. Or, if you already take them, it could help your medicines work better so you might be able to reduce the dose or take less tablets.

Eating a healthy balanced diet is not only important for your future health but can help make you feel much better in the short term too.

A BALANCED DIET
A healthy balanced diet includes:
● Plenty of fruit and vegetables – these should make up a third of your diet
● Plenty of starchy foods – these should make up another third of your diet
● Moderate amounts of lean meat, fish, eggs and other protein foods
● Moderate amounts of milk and dairy foods or dairy alternatives
● Limited amounts of food or drink high in salt, saturated fat or sugar

Here are some tips to help you achieve the right balance:

1 Eat at least five portions of fruit and veg every day
Fruit and vegetables are an important source of vitamins, minerals and other nutrients and can help protect against many diseases. They can also help to lower your blood pressure. Choose a variety of different types and colours for greatest benefits. See the section 'Eating More Fruit and Vegetables' for further advice.

2 Base your main meals on starchy foods
Starchy foods, also known as carbohydrates, include potatoes, plantain, yams, squash, bread, breakfast cereals, oats, pasta, rice and pulses such as lentils and chickpeas. They are a good source of energy, fibre, vitamins and minerals. Go for whole grain varieties when you can which usually have more nutrients and fibre.

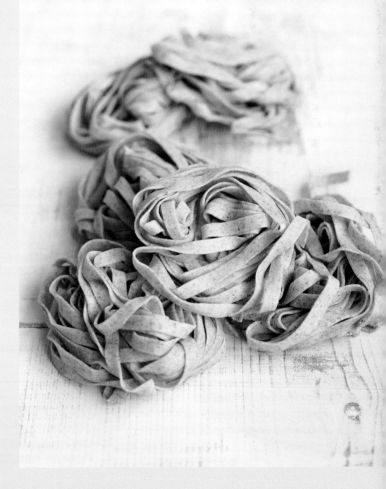

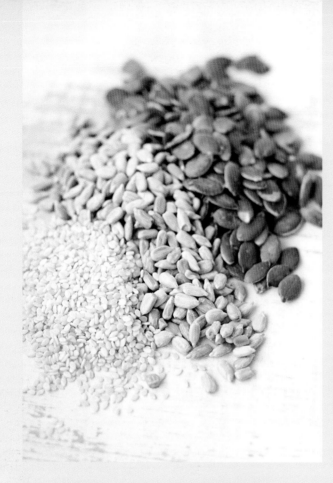

5 Eat less salt
Eating less salt can benefit everyone and is really important if you have high blood pressure. Adults should eat no more than six grams a day and children even less. The next few pages focus on eating less salt.

6 Eat less fat and limit foods high in saturated fat
Too much fat in the diet can lead to weight gain (it contains twice as many calories as protein or carbohydrate), and too much saturated fat raises your blood cholesterol, which increases your risk of heart disease. Try eating some foods high in unsaturated fats instead, such as oily fish, avocados, unsalted nuts and seeds as these can help lower cholesterol. See the final section 'Other Risk Factors' for more advice on fat.

7 Avoid added sugars in food and drinks
Cutting down on sugary foods and drinks may help you control your weight and is good for your teeth. As well as obviously sweet products, watch out for added sugars in many convenience foods.

8 Drink plenty of water or other fluids
In the UK, guidelines recommend that you around 1.2 litres of fluid (ideally water) every day, or more if you do a lot of exercise.

9 Enjoy healthy food
Healthy food can be enjoyable and tasty – the recipes in this book are proof of that!

3 Eat at least two portions of fish every week
Fish is a good source of protein, vitamins and minerals. The omega 3 fats found in oily fish may help prevent heart disease. Try to eat at least one portion of oily fish each week such as salmon, trout or mackerel (but no more than four portions a week, or no more than two portions if you are a woman who might have a child one day – see page 32).

4 Have some dairy (or dairy alternative) food every day
Milk and dairy are good sources of protein, vitamins and minerals and the best source of calcium in the diet, which can help keep bones strong. In the UK, there is no specific recommendation for how much dairy food to include in our diet but many dietitians advise we should eat three portions of a variety of lower-fat, reduced-salt versions every day in order to get enough calcium.

DASH AND MEDITERRANEAN DIETS

You may have read about the 'DASH' diet for lowering blood pressure and the 'Mediterranean' diet for reducing risk of heart disease. There is some interesting evidence to support these diets. Both are broadly similar to the principles of a healthy balanced diet outlined in this book, including lots of fruits, vegetables and whole grain foods. The DASH diet also emphasises cutting down on salt and eating low-fat dairy foods every day. And the Mediterranean diet includes olive oil (an unsaturated fat) as the main source of fat in the diet and moderate amounts of wine.

You do not need to follow a specific dietary plan to lower your blood pressure unless your doctor or nurse has advised you to. The key diet and lifestyle changes you can make to help lower your blood pressure are:

- Eat less salt (no more than six grams a day)
- Eat more fruit and vegetables (at least five portions)
- Lose weight if you need to
- Be more active (aim for thirty minutes five times a week)
- Drink alcohol in moderation (if at all)

DO I NEED SUPPLEMENTS?

Most people can get all the vitamins, minerals and other nutrients they need from a healthy balanced diet. There is currently no evidence to support the use of vitamin, mineral or herbal supplements to lower blood pressure. But if you do choose to take any and you also take blood pressure tablets, check first with your doctor because some supplements can cause unwanted effects of medicines in the body.

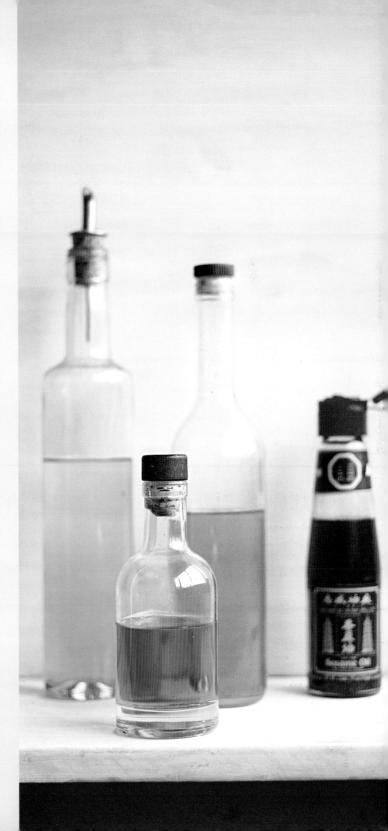

eating less salt

Most people in the UK eat too much salt. Adults should eat no more than six grams a day.

If you have high blood pressure, eating less salt is one of the best things you can do to help lower it. But even if you have normal blood pressure, cutting down on salt is a good strategy for helping you prevent high blood pressure as you get older. Eating less salt is important for the whole family.

SALT AND BLOOD PRESSURE
There is very good medical evidence that cutting down on salt will lower your blood pressure, whether you have high blood pressure or not.

How much salt should I eat?
The UK government has set a target of eating no more than six grams of salt a day. This is a realistic rather than ideal target because most people eat an average of nine grams or more. Some health professionals believe we should try to eat no more than three grams of salt a day which would have a much greater effect on lowering blood pressure.

Studies have found that if people with high blood pressure eat just three grams less salt a day they can lower their systolic pressure from between 3.6 to 5.6 mmHg and their diastolic pressure from between 1.9 to 3.2 mmHg. Eating six grams less salt a day would double this effect. This might not sound like a lot but any drop in blood pressure is a drop in your long term risk of stroke and heart disease. Over time you could see even bigger falls in blood pressure if you combine eating less salt with other diet and lifestyle changes.

'Salt sensitivity'
Everyone can benefit from eating less salt but some people seem to be especially sensitive to the effects of salt on their blood pressure. People of African-Caribbean origin, older people and those with a strong family history of high blood pressure seem to benefit even more than others from eating less salt. If this applies to you, eating a lot less than six grams of salt a day could make a really big difference to your blood pressure.

HOW TO CUT DOWN ON SALT
The problem with the UK diet is not so much about the salt we add at the table or use in cooking, although you should try to cut down on this. The bigger issue is that **around seventy five percent of the salt we eat is already in the food we buy.**

It can be difficult and time consuming to work out exactly how much salt you eat – you would need to weigh all your food and calculate the amount of salt in each item. Here are some easier, more practical ways to help you cut down:

1 Avoid or limit foods very high in salt
Some foods or ingredients are obviously salty such as:

- Prawns, anchovies, smoked or salted fish
- Smoked or processed meats like ham, bacon and tinned meat
- Stock cubes and gravy granules
- Olives
- Soy sauce
- Snacks like crisps, salted or dry roasted nuts
- Yeast extract

If you enjoy these foods it is not necessary to cut them out completely. Just try to save them for occasional treats on days when you will otherwise be mostly eating low salt foods. Or eat smaller amounts and look for low or reduced salt varieties.

2 Watch out for 'hidden salt'
Six grams may sound like a lot but it can be surprising how much salt is 'hidden' in food, quickly adding up to take you over six grams a day. One of the problems is that some foods containing salt do not taste obviously salty, for example:

- Bread, biscuits and bakery goods
- Some breakfast cereals
- Pre-packed lunch items like sandwiches, sushi and dressed salads
- Pesto, pasta and cooking sauces
- Pizzas and ready meals

Table 2 'Hidden' salt in everyday food and drink

	Portion size	Grams of salt per portion
Wholemeal bread	1 medium slice	0.5g
Digestive biscuits	2 biscuits	0.5g
Crumpets	1 crumpet	1g
Cinnamon and raisin bagels	1 bagel	0.8g
Carrot cake slices	1 slice (approx 25g)	0.25g
Bran flakes	1 average bowl (50g)	0.65g
Organic crispy rice cereal	1 average bowl (30g)	0.5g
Tomato ketchup	1 tablespoon (15ml)	0.5g
Reduced sugar / salt baked beans	Small can (200g)	1.1g
Medium cheddar	Small piece (30g)	0.5g
Sachet of instant hot chocolate	1 sachet as sold	0.3g

● Cheese (especially feta, edam, parmesan, blue and processed cheeses)
● Table sauces, pickles and salad dressings
● Some soups (fresh, tinned or packet)
● Instant food or drinks like noodles and hot chocolate
● Some brands of baked beans
● Takeaway food such as Chinese or Indian

Low salt	0.3g per 100g or less
Medium salt	more than 0.3g and up to 1.5g per 100g
High salt	more than 1.5g per 100g

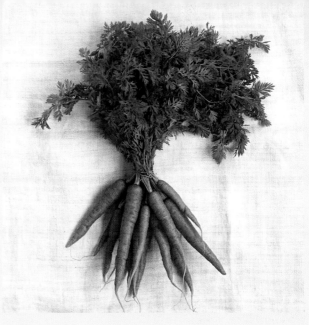

Take a look at table 2 for examples of how much salt is 'hidden' in some everyday products. Again, you do not need to cut out these foods altogether, especially bread, cereals and cheese which provide important nutrients. But simply being aware that they add salt to your diet can help you keep an eye on how much you are eating each day.

Many manufacturers are gradually reducing salt in foods sold in the UK. Quantities given here were accurate at the time of going to press, taken from UK product labels or website data.

3 Read the label

One easy way to cut down on salt is to check food labels and try to choose foods which are low in salt. Look at the amount of salt per 100g and use the following as a guide: You might find that some food labels list sodium instead of salt. Sodium is one part of salt (sodium chloride) and it is the sodium part that has an affect on blood pressure. Because sodium is also in other ingredients like monosodium glutamate and sodium bicarbonate, food labels have to give sodium rather than salt content per 100g.

If a label does not also give the amount of salt per 100g you can work it out yourself by assuming that 1g sodium = 2.5g salt. So where a product contains 0.5g sodium per 100g, multiply this by 2.5 to see it has roughly 1.25 grams salt per 100g.

Table 3 Salt savings: always check the label

Instead of...	Choose...	Salt you could save on...
½ pepperoni pizza	½ vegetable pizza	0.5g
Ready meal chicken biryani	Healthy version chicken biryani	2.8g
2 grilled pork sausages	1 grilled pork loin chop (150g)	1.75g
Crayfish and rocket sandwich	Poached salmon sandwich	1.1g
50g smoked salmon	1 plain salmon steak	1.5g
1 bowl of corn flakes (55g)	2 wheat biscuits	1g
1 breaded chicken breast fillet	1 plain skinless chicken breast	0.3g
2 rough oatcakes	2 rye crisp breads	0.4g
1 crumpet	1 scotch pancake	0.65g
30g edam cheese	30g reduced fat cheddar	0.3g
1 tablespoon tomato ketchup	1 tablespoon lower salt ketchup	0.2g
Cheese and onion crisps (35g)	Dried fruit and unsalted nuts (35g)	0.5g

Be aware that it is not just the amount of salt in a 100g of food that is important but the amount you eat too. If you are going to eat more than 100g of a food, look at the 'traffic light label' if there is one. The Food Standards Agency's recommended scheme takes account of the amount of saturated fat, salt and sugar per 100g and per serving – if the label is red ('high') for salt the product is best avoided or eaten in much smaller amounts.

4 Salt swaps
Comparing labels and swapping convenience foods for more natural foods is a good way to eat less salt. Take a look at table 3 to see how much salt you could save by making some straightforward food swaps.

5 Eat more natural foods and do not use salt in cooking
You can eat a lot less salt by replacing processed foods with your own meals made with fresh and natural ingredients (with no added salt) – try some of the recipes in this book.

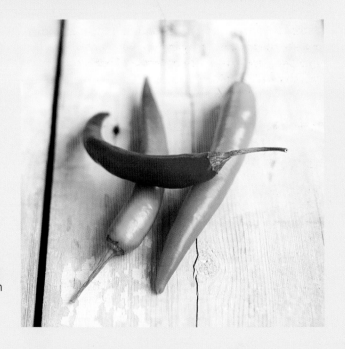

Eating this way is not only better for you but can be so much more tasty and satisfying too. When you cook there are many different ways you can flavour food instead of using salt or salty ingredients. For example, try using:

● Pepper, garlic, onions, chillies, lemon juice, fresh ginger, vinegar, herbs and spices

But be aware that some curry powders, spice and herb mixes have added salt – check the label to be sure they are salt free.

6 Get used to the taste of less salt

Enjoying food which tastes very salty is purely from habit. If you cut down on salt you could be surprised how quickly your taste buds adapt. You may even find after a few weeks you no longer like the taste of the salty foods you used to enjoy.

7 Children should eat less salt too

The amount of salt children should eat is even less than adults. Table 4 shows the recommended daily limits of salt for children of different ages.

Babies below the age of one need only a tiny amount of salt – their kidneys cannot cope with more than 1g a day. For more advice on feeding babies see www.eatwell.gov.uk.

Key points
● Eating less salt can help your lower blood pressure
● Eat no more than six grams of salt a day – children should have even less
● Watch out for 'hidden' salt – seventy five per cent is already in the food we buy
● Read food labels – choose foods with less salt
● Eat more natural foods – they usually have less salt than processed foods
● Start to enjoy the taste of less salt – your taste buds will quickly adapt

There is good evidence that what children eat in early life influences their food choices when they are adults. If you encourage your children to eat less salt from an early age they are more likely to enjoy the taste of a lower salt diet when they are older. This will put them at lower risk of developing high blood pressure in the future.

Watch out for breakfast cereals, snack products and other processed foods aimed at children which are often high in salt. Remember that children's favourites like tomato ketchup and sausages can also add a lot of salt to their diet.

Table 4 Maximum salt intake for children

Age	No more than...
1 to 3 years	2g per day
4 to 6 years	3g per day
7 to 10 years	5g per day
11 and over	6g per day

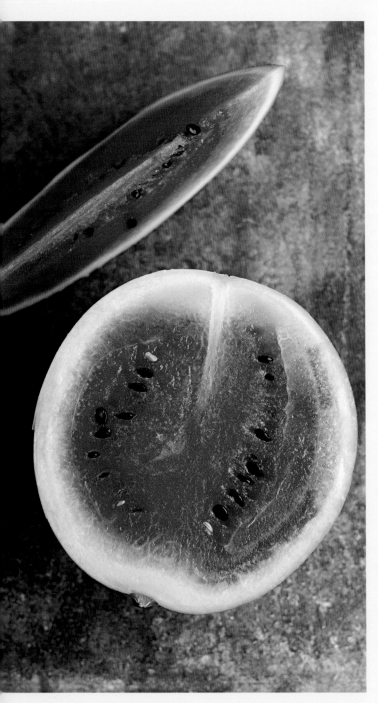

eating more fruit and vegetables

We should all be trying to eat at least five portions of a variety of fruit and vegetables every day. But most people in the UK eat less than three portions a day.

There are many good reasons to eat lots of fruit and vegetables. There is good evidence for example that eating at least five portions a day can lower your risk of diabetes, obesity, stroke, heart disease and some types of cancer. Eating lots of fruit and vegetables can also help lower your blood pressure. They are a very good source of potassium, a mineral that has the reverse effect in the body to salt. By eating at least five portions a day you will help your body get all the potassium it needs.

As well as protecting your future health you can gain instant benefits from eating more fruit and vegetables. They are mostly low in fat and calories so can help you control your weight. And because of all the important vitamins, minerals, fibre and other nutrients they contain, eating more fruit and vegetables can boost your energy and help you feel better every day.

A handful of grapes
2 or more smaller fruits e.g. 2 plums, 2 satsumas, 3 fresh dates, 7 strawberries
1 medium fruit e.g. apple, orange, banana, pear
½ large fruit e.g. avocado, grapefruit*
1 large slice of a large fruit e.g. melon, papaya, pineapple
1 tablespoon of dried fruit e.g. raisins
1 glass (150ml) of 100% fruit or vegetable juice or smoothie
3 heaped tablespoons of vegetables or cooked pulses
1 cereal bowl of mixed salad leaves
1 medium fresh tomato or 7 cherry tomatoes
Half a pepper

Table 5 Example portion sizes

* Grapefruit juice can effect the action of some medicines – ask your doctor if you should avoid it, especially if you take statins or calcium channel blockers. Other fruit juices are fine.

WHAT IS A PORTION?

A portion is roughly 80g of the edible part of a fruit or vegetable, not including the core or peel, or around 150ml of pure juice. Table 5 gives examples of what counts as a portion. You can find a more detailed list on the 5 A Day website: www.5aday.nhs.uk.

WHY '5 A DAY'?

Around twenty years ago the World Health Organisation (WHO) first set the recommendation to eat more fruit and vegetables. This came from studies that found that healthy populations ate around 400 grams or more of fruit and vegetables (excluding potatoes) every day.

Since a portion of fruit or vegetable is roughly 80 grams, five portions adds up to roughly 400 grams – this is where the '5 A Day' message came from. But many health professionals now believe we should try to eat more than 400 grams a day so some countries have changed their health messages to reflect this.

Can supplements provide the same benefits?

Studies that have looked at taking nutrient supplements (vitamins and minerals for example) have mostly concluded they do not have the same beneficial effects as eating fruit and vegetables. It appears that fruit and vegetables have a unique mix of vitamins, minerals, fibre and other nutrients that work together to protect our health in a way that supplements cannot replicate.

5 A DAY: WHAT COUNTS

All fresh, frozen, chilled, tinned and dried fruit and vegetables count. Fruit and vegetables found in dishes like soup, stews and convenience foods also count but it is best to avoid those with a lot of added salt, saturated fat or sugar.

Variety is important

Different fruit and vegetables provide a different mix of vitamins, minerals, antioxidants and other nutrients. So it is important to try to eat a variety of different types each day.

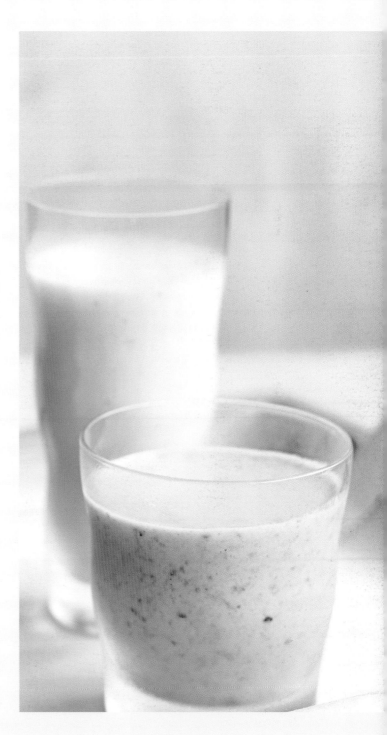

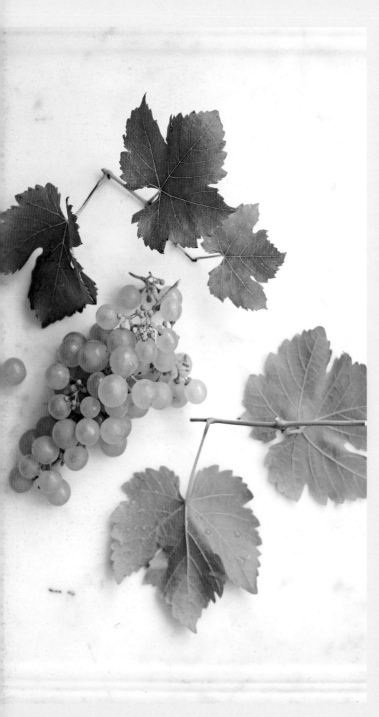

Juice, smoothies and pulses

100% fruit or vegetable juice and smoothies can count towards your 5 A Day. But fruit juice can only count as one of your portions per day no matter how much you drink. This is because fruit juice contains less of the beneficial nutrients found in whole fruit such as fibre, and the high levels of natural sugars in juice can be bad for your teeth. The same applies to pulses such as lentils and chickpeas. These can count towards your 5 A Day but again only as one portion a day. Remember that pulses also count as starchy foods which are an important part of a healthy balanced diet.

Potatoes do not count!

Potatoes and other starchy root vegetables like cassava, yams and plantain do not count towards 5 A Day. They are of course vegetables but because they are an important source of carbohydrate in the diet they count as starchy foods instead.

CHILDREN SHOULD EAT MORE TOO

There are no specific guidelines in the UK on portion sizes for children but they should be encouraged to eat a variety of fruit and vegetables every day. This will help them develop a taste for them and make them more likely to eat fruit and vegetables as they grow up, helping to protect their future health.

TIPS ON GETTING YOUR 5 A DAY

5 A Day may sound a lot to achieve but it's surprising how easy it can be to make it a healthy new habit. If you have one or two portions at each main meal and snack on fresh fruit you can easily reach your five or more portions a day.

Here are a few ideas to help you eat more fruit and vegetables:

● Add fruit to your cereal or porridge – try sliced banana, apple or fresh or frozen berries
● Blend any fruit you like with a touch of juice or low-fat yogurt for a healthy smoothie
● Snack on raw vegetable sticks with reduced fat hummus
● Add lettuce and tomatoes to your lunchtime sandwich

- Add vegetables, lentils or beans to stews or casseroles
- Make fresh soups or stir fries using lots of vegetables

GETTING THE MOST FROM YOUR FRUIT AND VEG

To get the most from fruit and vegetables try to:
- Choose mostly natural fruit and vegetables – convenience foods such as vegetable curries, tinned fruit or ready-to-roast vegetables often have lots of added salt, fat or sugar
- Buy fresh fruit and vegetables in season and grown locally – they are likely to contain more vitamins
- Eat lots of different coloured fruit and vegetables each day to get the best range of nutrients
- Choose tinned or frozen fruit and vegetables without added sugar or salt

Preparing and cooking vegetables
The way you prepare and cook vegetables can affect the amount of vitamins left in them and their salt, fat and calorie content. Here are some tips to help preserve vitamins and keep your vegetables healthy:

- Steam vegetables when possible
- Chop vegetables immediately before cooking – do not leave them sitting in water
- Eat vegetables as soon as they have been cooked
- If you boil vegetables cut them into larger chunks and cook in as little water and for as short a time as possible
- If you fry or roast vegetables do not add oil or use just a tiny amount of an unsaturated oil (such as olive oil) – vegetables absorb fat during cooking
- Avoid adding salt to vegetables when cooking or serving them – try pepper or herbs instead

Key points
- Eating more fruit and vegetables can help lower your blood pressure
- Fruit and vegetables help protect against a range of diseases
- Eat at least five portions a day – aim to eat a variety of different types and colours

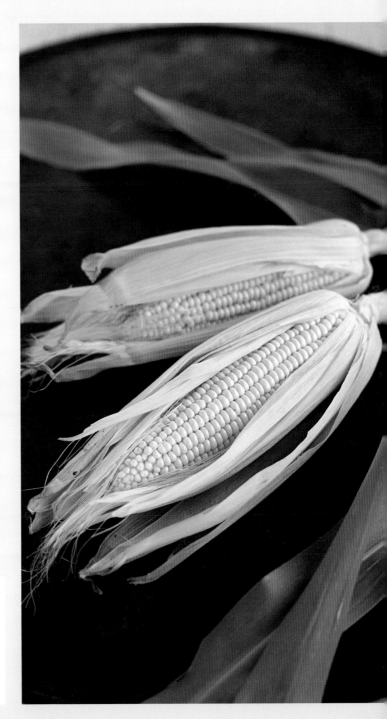

healthy weight

Around three in five adults in the UK are above their ideal weight. Being overweight puts a strain on your heart and can increase your blood pressure. Losing weight if you need to is a very effective way to lower your blood pressure and has other important health benefits too.

Losing weight is not always easy. A huge industry has built up around dieting which tries to tempt us with quick fix solutions to losing weight. But while some 'fad' diets may seem to work in the short term, most people quickly put the weight back on when they go back to their usual eating habits.

The key to losing weight and keeping it off is to make small, gradual changes to what you eat that you can keep up for life, and to be more active if you can.

DO I NEED TO LOSE WEIGHT?
If you are not sure if you could benefit from losing weight you can use waist and body mass index (BMI) measurements as useful guides.

Waist measurement
Your waist measurement is a measure of how much fat you carry around your middle – if you carry excess fat here you are more likely to suffer health problems from being overweight.

You can measure your waist with a tape measure. Place it round your midriff roughly at the level of your tummy button. You are at more risk of developing health problems if your waist measures:

- Women: 80 cm or above
- Men: 94 cm or above

Body Mass Index (BMI)
The BMI is a guide to whether you are the right weight for your height. To work it out you can use one of the many BMI calculators found on the internet (try www.eatwell.gov.uk). Or use the following equation: BMI = weight (kilograms) / height (metres) x height (metres).

The following is a guide to what your BMI means:
BMI less than 18.5: underweight
BMI between 18.5 and 24.9: healthy weight
BMI between 25 and 29.9: overweight
BMI of 30 or above: obese

If your BMI is 25 or more you are at increased risk of health problems. And the more overweight you are the greater the risks. If your BMI is 35 or above you may need specialist help to manage your weight and health – visit your GP or nurse for advice.

However, the BMI applies only to adults and is not the best measurement for everyone. For example it is not suitable for those with well developed muscles such as athletes.

If you are of South Asian origin and living in the UK you should aim for a lower BMI and lower waist measurement than given above – your doctor or nurse can advise you. This is because you are at greater risk of developing diabetes and heart disease than the general UK population.

BENEFITS OF LOSING WEIGHT
There are many good reasons to lose weight if you need to. For example, it can help:

- Lower your blood pressure
- Reduce your risk of stroke, heart disease and some types of cancer
- Manage your diabetes (or reduce your risk of developing it)
- Improve back and joint pain
- Improve your sleep
- Improve your mood
- Improve your fertility
- Boost your energy so you can enjoy life to the full

Have a think about why you want to lose weight. For example, would you like to have more energy or less joint pain so you can play with your grandchildren? It is a good idea to write down your reasons for wanting to lose weight. They can act as a reminder when you are finding it tough to keep going.

HOW TO LOSE WEIGHT

If you are overweight you have taken in more calories (energy) from food and drink over the years than your body has used up. To lose weight you need to reverse this.

Successful and long term weight loss means making sensible and healthy changes to your diet (so you eat less calories) and being more active (so you use up more calories). See the next section for advice on being more active.

Here are some tips to get you started:

1 Set yourself a realistic goal

It is important to set yourself a goal that is achievable so you are less likely to be disappointed and give up. Health experts believe that losing five to ten per cent of your body weight is a realistic target to aim for. This can bring about positive health benefits such as lower blood pressure.

2 Take it slowly

Those who lose weight slowly, say one to two pounds (0.5 to 1 kg) each week, tend to be more successful at losing weight and keeping it off. If you lose weight more quickly you might be losing muscle rather than fat which is not a healthy way to lose weight.

Each pound of body fat contains roughly 3,500 calories. To lose a pound a week you need to eat 500 calories less a day or be more active and use up 500 calories more a day (or ideally a combination of the two).

Making small and gradual changes to what you eat and being more active can really add up to make a big difference to your weight over time.

3 Try not to think of it as 'going on a diet'

Try not to get too obsessed with food or think of it as 'going on a diet'. Focus instead on achieving a healthy balance in your diet. This way you can take in fewer calories overall by eating lots of fruit and vegetables and whole grain starchy foods and cutting down on high fat and sugar foods which contain a lot of calories.

It can take a lot of time and effort to lose weight. What you eat every single day is not so important as how much you eat in total over the weeks and months ahead.

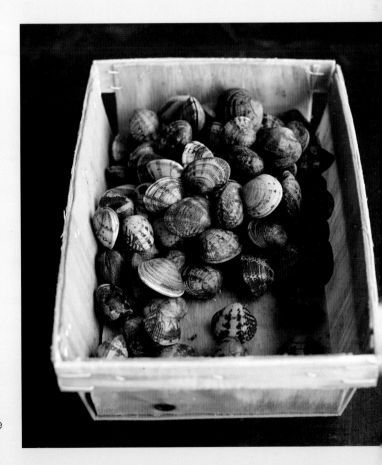

4 Do not restrict food groups

Some popular diets encourage you to cut out whole food groups like carbohydrates (starchy foods). Any diet that restricts fruit, vegetables or whole grain starchy foods is not a healthy way to lose weight – you will not get the full range of nutrients you need.

The reason most people lose weight on these 'fad' diets is that they simply eat less than they usually would. You can get the same effect in a much more healthy way by eating a balanced diet with less fat and sugar and by being more active.

5 Get some support

Some people feel they need an eating plan to help them lose weight or the support of others. It is a good idea to visit your GP or practice nurse – they can let you know of support available in your area, for example if there is a dietitian who could help you or a local support group.

Commercial slimming clubs are helpful for some people. But remember the goal is to make small, lifelong changes to your diet – check that a club offers help on how to stop putting weight back on in the long term, not just how to lose it.

If you do not enjoy being in a group there are many websites with information and tools to help you stay motivated including:

www.nationalobesityforum.org.uk
www.eatwell.gov.uk
www.weightconcern.org.uk
www.bdaweightwise.com
www.weightlossresources.co.uk

SMALL CHANGES ADD UP

Small changes you make to your diet and activity levels can really add up over the months ahead to help you lose weight and keep it off. Here are some tips on changes you could make to help you lose weight the healthy way:

Control your appetite

● Do not skip breakfast – research shows it helps people maintain a healthy weight
● Eat at regular times during the day to avoid overeating if you get too hungry
● Go for brown or wholegrain foods with lots of fibre which are more filling
● Have some protein with main meals such as lean meat, fish, eggs, lentils or beans
● Be careful if you drink alcohol – it can make you feel more hungry and adds calories too
● Drink plenty of water – being dehydrated can be mistaken for hunger

Eat less fat

● Choose reduced fat dairy foods such as semi-skimmed milk and lower fat spreads
● Remove visible fat or skin from meat before cooking
● Grill, poach, steam, bake or dry roast instead of frying or roasting in oil

Other ways to cut calories

● Plan meals and snacks ahead of time so you always have healthy food at hand
● Compare food labels of similar products – go for those with less calories
● Reduce your portion sizes – try using smaller plates and bowls if it helps
● Pile up your plate with vegetables – they are filling and low in calories
● Replace high calories snacks with fresh fruit
● Drink less sugary drinks

Key points
● Losing weight if you need to is an effective way to lower your blood pressure
● Losing weight has many other positive benefits for your health and wellbeing
● The best way to lose weight is to make lifelong changes to what you eat and be more active

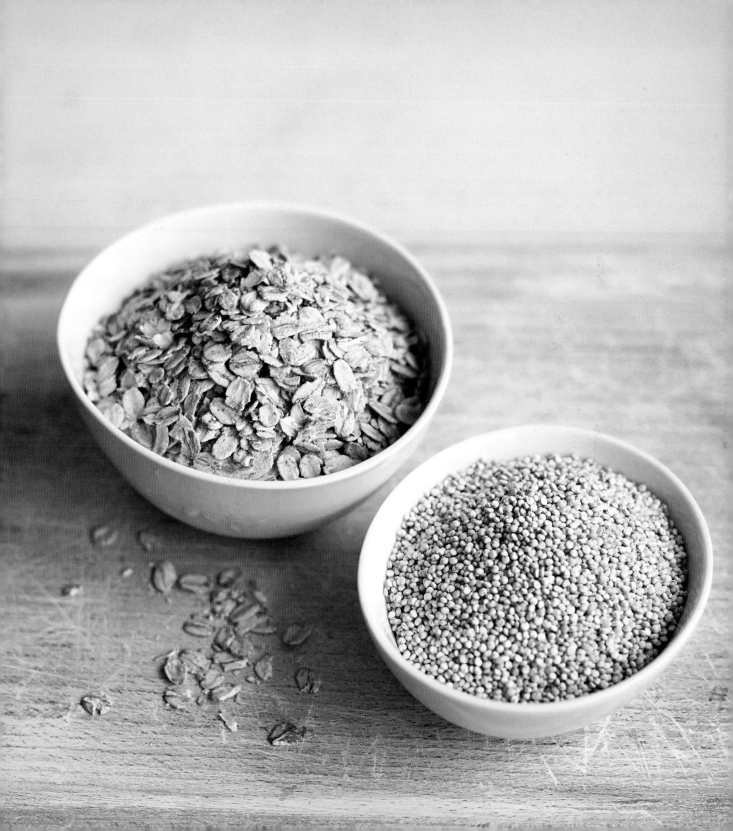

being active

The majority of adults in the UK do not do enough physical activity. Being inactive can have a major, negative impact on your health.

Adults who are physically active have around a thirty per cent reduced risk of premature death and up to a fifty per cent reduced risk of developing heart disease, stroke, diabetes, some types of cancer and other illnesses.

In the short term being more active can help to lower your blood pressure and improve your cholesterol levels. It can also help you sleep better, have more energy, feel less stressed and reduce your risk of depression and anxiety. And being more active is one of the best ways to lose weight and keep it off when combined with a healthy balanced diet.

What is an active lifestyle?

The UK government recommends 'at least five a week' for adults. This means doing thirty minutes of at least 'moderate intensity' activity on five or more days of the week. Moderate intensity means any activity that gets you warm and makes you breathe a bit faster.

Whatever your age, young or old, being more active in your day to day life can make you feel better and lowers your risk of health problems in the future.

ACTIVITY AND BLOOD PRESSURE

Exercise causes a temporary rise in blood pressure and when you stop exercising your blood pressure should return to its usual resting levels. But in the long term being more active can help to reduce your blood pressure levels overall.

It is a good idea to check how safe it is for you to take up any new activity, especially if you are new to exercise or have just been diagnosed with high blood pressure. Your doctor or nurse can advise. If you have very high blood pressure (200/110 or above) always check first.

If you have high blood pressure you should avoid any type of exercise that causes a quick rise in your blood pressure or places strain on your heart. This includes weight lifting, sprinting and playing squash. Scuba diving and parachuting can also be dangerous – always check with your doctor first.

WHAT IS THE BEST TYPE OF EXERCISE?

Unless you enjoy it you do not need to do strenuous gym workouts or take up running. It is better to try to fit some activity into your daily routine that you enjoy and will keep up in the long term. For example, you could walk or cycle to work instead of driving. Or take up an active hobby like bowling, dancing, or gardening.

You can do your thirty minutes of activity in bouts of ten minutes or more. For example three ten minute walks in a day could have as much benefit as one thirty minute walk. Build up gradually until activity becomes a normal part of your daily routine.

Exercise that is good for your heart

High blood pressure is a risk factor for heart disease. So if you have high blood pressure it makes sense for you to do the types of exercise that can improve the condition of your heart and blood vessels. This means doing some aerobic exercise that gets you a little out of breath such as brisk walking, jogging, dancing or swimming.

Exercise that is good for your bones

It is a good idea to also do some weight-bearing exercise to help protect your bones. In young adults this helps maintain the density and strength of bones. In older adults it helps to slow the loss of bone that tends to happen with age – this helps prevent osteoporosis, a condition which increases the risk of broken bones.

Weight-bearing exercise includes brisk walking, skipping, dancing, aerobics, playing tennis or jogging, or any other activity where you support the weight of your own body.

Activities for older people

It is important to remain active when you are older. Activities that help build your strength, coordination and balance can help you maintain your mobility, independence and ability to do everyday tasks. It can also help reduce your risk of falling and getting injured.

To avoid injury you should avoid higher intensity activities or any activity which involves sudden or complicated movements, unless you are used to these types of exercise.

Exercise and mobility

If you are unable to get up unaided from a chair you could ask your doctor or nurse about chair-based exercise classes in your area. These can help you gently build up your fitness.

HOW TO BE MORE ACTIVE

Here are some ideas to help you get more active for life:

● Take up an active hobby like golf or bowls
● Find a 'gym buddy' – having a friend to exercise with can make it more fun
● Schedule a walk into your daily routine, for example walk around the block at lunchtime
● Find a local 'green gym' to get active at the same time as helping the environment – see www.btcv.org.uk for information
● Join a Ramblers weekly walking group – they have groups for different ages and abilities – see www.ramblers.org.uk
● Get an allotment – gardening is a good way to keep active
● Yoga, T'ai Chi and pilates can keep you supple and help your posture and balance – most local sports centres now offer classes
● Remember that everyday activities such as housework and climbing stairs count too

Key points

● Being active helps lower blood pressure and reduces your risk of other health problems
● Aim to be active for at least thirty minutes on five days of the week
● Aim for moderate intensity activity which gets you a bit warm and a little out of breath
● To keep your heart healthy try to fit in some aerobic exercise
● Being active is important for all ages, young or old

alcohol

Drinking too much alcohol increases your risk of high blood pressure and other health problems too. In the UK nearly one in three men and one in five women drink too much alcohol. In other words they regularly drink more than the recommended daily limit of:

● Three to four units a day for men
● Two to three units a day for women

Limits for women are lower because of their smaller body size and different body composition, with more fat and less water to dilute alcohol. It is advisable for pregnant women, or those trying to get pregnant, to avoid alcohol altogether.

Benefits of moderate alcohol consumption

For many of us drinking alcohol is a normal part of our lives and there can be some benefits to drinking it. It can help you relax and unwind for example. And drinking moderate amounts (one or two units a day) seems to protect against heart disease in men over the age of forty and post-menopausal women. But that is not to say you should drink alcohol to protect your heart – eating a healthy diet, being active and giving up smoking can bring about much greater benefits.

Risks of regular over-drinking

People who drink too much alcohol tend to have raised blood pressure. Regularly drinking more than is recommended also increases the risk of other health problems like stroke, heart and liver disease, and probably raises the risk of mental health problems like depression and anxiety. Alcohol also increases the risk of some types of cancer including mouth and breast cancer.

If you do choose to drink alcohol it is important to stay within recommended limits to help keep your blood pressure levels healthy and reduce your risk of future ill health.

BENEFITS OF CUTTING DOWN

Most people who suffer health problems from alcohol are not alcoholics. Rather they are people who regularly drink more than is recommended over a number of years. This causes a build-up of damage in the body over time, resulting in health problems in the long term.

You can gain many short and long term benefits from cutting down on alcohol if you regularly drink more than is recommended. For example, it could:

● Lower your blood pressure and risk of stroke
● Reduce your risk of some types of cancer and other diseases
● Help you feel better and improve your mental wellbeing
● Improve your sleep
● Give you better skin
● Boost your fertility
● Help you lose weight if you need to
● Improve your sex life – alcohol can cause temporary impotence in men

UNITS OF ALCOHOL

It is important to be aware that the strengths of many alcoholic drinks, for example wine and lager, have increased in recent years, as have serving sizes. Because of this it is easy to underestimate how much you drink. Table 6 gives examples of some alcoholic drinks and the number of units they contain.

Many alcoholic drinks now include a label to let you know how many units they contain. Or you could work out how many units you are drinking by using the 'units calculator' on the NHS website: units.nhs.uk/unitCalculator.html.

Table 6

Type of drink	No of Units
Single gin (40%) and tonic	1 unit
175ml (standard glass) red, white or rose wine (13%)	2.3 units
1 pint of lager (4%)	2.3 units
1 pint of lager (5%)	2.8 units
1 pint of bitter (4%)	2.3 units
½ bottle of wine (13%)	5 units
1 alcopop (5%)	1.4 units

BINGE DRINKING

You have probably seen a lot of media coverage on the 'binge drinking' culture in the UK. Binge drinking means reaching a state of intoxication on any one drinking session.

There is no specific definition on binge drinking. But roughly it means drinking more than six units of alcohol in any one session for women, or more than eight for men. If you look at table 6 and the number of units in many drinks, you can see how easy it can be to exceed these amounts – a woman drinking just three glasses of a standard pub glass of wine (175ml) could be having more than six units if the wine is of a higher strength (13%).

Binge drinking is particularly bad for health as it can greatly increase blood pressure in the short term and risk of stroke. It is much better to stay within the maximum daily limits of alcohol units than to 'save them up' for one or two heavy drinking sessions. This is why the government now recommends a daily maximum number of units rather than the old weekly maximum.

TIPS FOR CUTTING DOWN

If you think you should try to drink less, here are some practical ways to do this:

- Aim to have a few alcohol free days each week
- Try low alcohol options like low strength beer
- Alternate alcoholic drinks with water or low-cal soft drink
- Dilute drinks like white wine with water or soda
- Sip your drink slowly and drink lots of water to keep hydrated
- Avoid salty snacks when drinking – they make you thirsty so you are likely to drink more
- If you drink too much alcohol wait 48 hours before having any more to help your body recover

If you think that you, a friend or family member might have a problem with alcohol, you could visit your GP for advice. There are also many organisations offering help and advice in the UK including:

Alcoholics Anonymous: www.al-anonuk.org.uk

Alcohol Concern: www.alcoholconcern.org.uk

Key points
- Drinking alcohol is a personal choice and moderate drinking can have positive health benefits
- Women should drink no more than 2 to 3 units a day; men no more than 3 to 4 units a day
- Drinking too much alcohol can increase your blood pressure and risk of other health problems
- Binge drinking is especially bad for your blood pressure and health

other risk factors

Coronary heart disease (CHD) is the name given to the gradual narrowing of blood vessels in the body that can lead to angina and heart attacks. It is the single most common cause of death in the UK.

High blood pressure is one of the major risk factors for CHD.

Other known risk factors include:

Factors you cannot change
- Getting older
- Gender (men are at greater risk at an earlier age)
- Family history
- Ethnicity (South Asian people in the UK are more at risk of CHD)

Factors you can change or manage
- High blood pressure
- High cholesterol
- Smoking
- Diabetes
- Obesity
- Physical inactivity
- Drinking too much alcohol

If you have more than one risk factor your risk of CHD is much increased. So if you have high blood pressure it makes sense for you to keep your cholesterol levels healthy and to stop smoking too, as well as making the diet and lifestyle changes already outlined in this book.

CHOLESTEROL

High levels of cholesterol in your blood increases your risk of developing CHD and stroke. Diet and lifestyle factors play a major role in your risk of developing high cholesterol as well as its treatment.

Cholesterol and heart disease

There are several types of cholesterol in the body. Scientists believe that the two main types related to risk of heart disease are High Density Lipoprotein (HDL) and Low Density Lipoprotein (LDL). If you have high levels of LDL (also known as 'bad cholesterol') this can lead to narrowing and blockage of your blood vessels which could eventually lead to a heart attack, stroke or other complications.

Higher levels of HDL cholesterol (also known as 'good cholesterol') seem to be protective against heart disease. The reasons are not yet clear but low levels of HDL seem to be an important risk factor for heart disease in European and North American adults. Being physically active can help increase your HDL cholesterol levels.

There is another type of fat in the blood called triglyceride. If you have high triglyceride levels and low HDL cholesterol you are at higher risk of CHD. Obesity is a major cause of this. Losing weight and being more active can help reverse this risk factor.

Healthy cholesterol

The only way to know if your cholesterol levels are healthy is to have a blood test. If you have high blood pressure or any other risk factors for heart disease it is a good idea to ask your doctor, nurse or pharmacist for a cholesterol check.

If your cholesterol levels are on the high side of normal or they are too high, it is likely your doctor or nurse will ask you to make some changes to your diet and lifestyle. Your doctor might also prescribe cholesterol lowering medicines.

CHANGING YOUR DIET TO LOWER CHOLESTEROL

Eating a balanced diet with lots of fruit and vegetables and whole grain starchy foods can help keep your cholesterol levels healthy. Other lifestyle factors like being physically active, not smoking, keeping to a healthy weight and not drinking too much alcohol are also very important.

Other specific aspects of your diet you can change to help lower your cholesterol levels include:

1 Eat less saturated fat

Some cholesterol is already in foods we eat such as liver or eggs. But the much greater problem is the cholesterol made in our bodies from the saturated fat in our diet. Cutting down on saturated fat is very important for lowering your cholesterol and keeping it at healthy levels.

Animal fats, coconut and palm oil are all sources of saturated fat. Foods that tend to be high in saturated fat include:
- Fatty cuts of meat
- Processed meats
- Butter, ghee, lard
- Full fat dairy foods
- Pastries, cakes, biscuits
- Snacks and chocolate

Eating less of these foods will help you cut down on saturated fat. Try to also avoid eating visible fat or skin on meat, and swap full fat dairy foods for reduced fat versions.

Food labels

You can also cut down on saturated fat by comparing food labels and trying to choose products with a low amount of saturated fat (or eat much smaller amounts of foods with a high amount). Look at the amount of 'saturates' or 'sat fat' per 100g and use the following as a guide:

Low saturated fat	1.5g per 100g or less
Medium saturated fat	more than 1.5g and up to 5g per 100g
High saturated fat	more than 5g per 100g

Another quick and simple way to eat less saturated fat is to use 'traffic light labels' on products when available. Try to avoid products that are labelled red for saturated fat – these contain a high amount.

2 Include some unsaturated fat in your diet

Unsaturated fats (including polyunsaturated and monounsaturated oils) can help reduce cholesterol levels and lower your risk of heart disease.

Foods that contain unsaturated fats include:

- Oily fish (see below)
- Avocados
- Nuts and seeds
- Sunflower oil
- Rapeseed and olive oil
- Spreads made with mono- or polyunsaturated oils

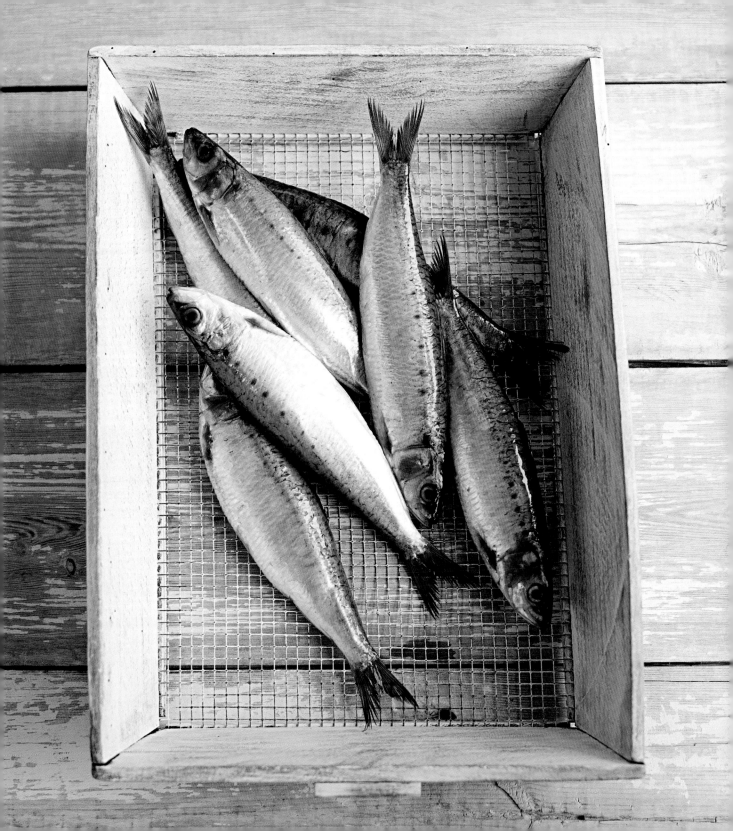

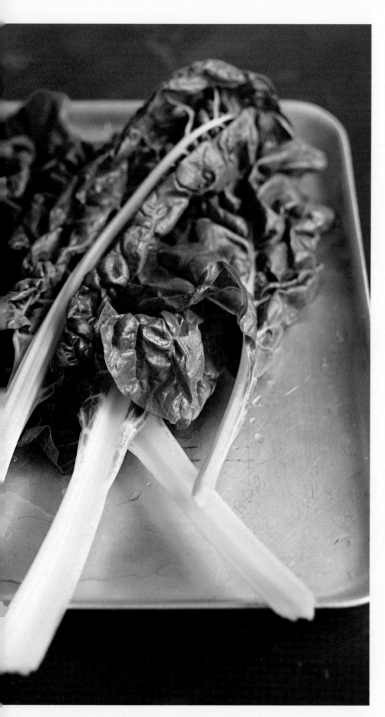

3 Eat more oily fish

Oily fish is the best source of omega 3 fat, a type of unsaturated fat that can lower triglyceride levels and help prevent heart disease. Oily fish includes salmon, trout, mackerel, sardines and herring. Try to eat at least one portion a week.

Sustainability of fish stocks is an important environmental issue – try to choose sustainably sourced fish when you can. To find out more see the Marine Stewardship Council's website at: www.msc.org

There are limits on how much oily fish we should eat due to environmental pollutants that build up in them. Boys, men and women who will not have a child in the future can eat up to four portions a week. Girls or women who are pregnant, breastfeeding or might have a child one day should have no more than two portions a week. You can find more information on recommended limits in the UK and further advice on oily fish and pregnant women on the Food Standards Agency website at: www.eatwell.gov.uk.

Research indicates that omega 3 fats found in vegetable sources like flaxseed (linseed) oil do not have the same beneficial effects as those from oily fish. They can still be included as part of a healthy diet and may be a useful alternative for vegetarians not wishing to take fish oils.

4 Eat foods high in soluble fibre

Soluble fibre in the diet can help lower cholesterol levels. Soluble fibre is found in:

● Oats
● Pulses like lentils and beans
● Some fruits and vegetables

5 Use products fortified with plant sterols or stanols

You could try having foods with added plant sterols or stanols. HEART UK (the UK's cholesterol charity: www.heartuk.org.uk) advises eating three portions a day of spreads, yoghurts or milk fortified with these to help lower your cholesterol. Eating between 2 to 2.5g per day of sterols or stanols can help achieve a cholesterol lowering effect of ten to fifteen per cent.

smoking and heart disease

One in five deaths from CHD is associated with smoking. Smokers are at much greater risk of having a heart attack than non-smokers. Stopping smoking is the single best thing you can do to avoid a future heart attack and prevent other diseases like lung cancer.

It is never too late to give up smoking. Visit your doctor or nurse to find out about services available locally to help you quit. Or there are many organisations in the UK that can offer advice and support on stopping smoking including:

NHS smokefree website: http://smokefree.nhs.uk
(Free helpline – 0800 022 4 332)
Quit: www.quit.org.uk (Quitline – 0800 00 22 00)
British Heart Foundation: www.bhf.org.uk/smoking
(Free Smoking Advice Line – 0800 169 1900)

To summarise the changes you can make to lower your blood pressure and reduce your risk of a future heart attack, stroke or other health problems:

1 Eat less salt: no more than six grams a day (much less is better)
2 Eat more fruit and vegetables: at least five portions of a variety every day
3 Lose weight if you need to: make small changes to your diet that you can keep up for life
4 Be more active: aim for thirty minutes at least five times a week
5 Drink alcohol sensibly: no more than 2 to 3 units a day for women; 3 to 4 units a day for men
6 Eat oily fish: at least one portion a week
7 Lower your cholesterol: eat less saturated fat, more unsaturated fat and some soluble fibre
8 If you smoke: seek help to quit

Remember, small steps can lead to big changes in the months and years ahead that can lower your blood pressure and dramatically reduce your risk of health problems in the future.

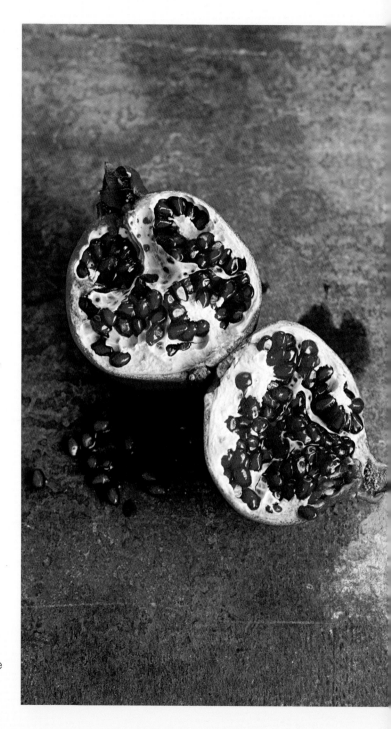

essential equipment

A kitchen with the following equipment will not only encourage a healthier style of cooking but also, in turn, make the job easier and your results more successful.

Always buy the best-quality equipment you can afford. It will do the job better and should last a lot longer too.

● Good-quality heavy-based pans of varying sizes. In general, I suggest using non-stick pans as they allow you to reduce the amount of fat you use in cooking without causing food to stick. You also need frying pans, including deep-sided for braising, which are suitable for oven use.

● A pan grill or flat griddle for grilling. There are some special low-fat grills on the market now that drain away the cooking fat. In the summer, take advantage of your barbecue char grill unit as it will cook vegetables and meat in particular with incredible flavour.

● Heavy-based casserole dishes or similar ovenproof dishes with lids for braising and stewing.

● Good-quality deep-sided non-stick woks for low-fat stir-frying, which enable you to use very little fat when cooking.

● Non-stick roasting tins of varying sizes.

● Non-stick baking tins and flat baking trays.

● Small steamer unit (or small Chinese steamer baskets).

● A centrifugal juice extractor is one of my favourite pieces of equipment; brilliant for extracting the maximum juice from fruit and vegetables as well as retaining healthy vitamins.

healthy cooking methods for healthy eating

When you are trying to establish healthy eating habits, how you cook your food is just as important as what food you eat.

The cooking methods described below are the best for retaining flavour, nutrients and good all-round health.

GRILLING
Grilling is a fast and extremely healthy way to cook, as it uses minimum fat in the process.

Using a preheated pan grill or outdoor char grill, gives a delicious smoky flavour to foods. Alternatively, use a grill rack placed under a conventional grill.

By marinating in advance or using an oil-water spray foods can be grilled using little or no fat.

ROASTING / DRY-ROASTING
Roasting is a cooking method that uses dry heat in an oven. Buy the leanest possible meat available for roasting and cook food on a wire rack inside a roasting tin so that any fat drains away during cooking.

I advise using non-stick roasting tins, thereby using minimal fat at all times.

Meats, fish and vegetables are delicious roasted and roasting helps retain valuable nutrients in the food, like vitamins.

Dry-roasting is usually reserved for such foods as nuts, spices and seeds.flavour to the food.

Herbs may also be added to foods as they roast, adding flavour to the food.

BAKING
This is another excellent healthy cooking method, great for cooking smaller pieces of fish and vegetables, as well as fruits. Again I suggest using non-stick baking tins for the job.

STEAMING
One of the healthiest and simplest ways to cook low fat dishes, as foods require no fat. Food is placed in a perforated basket and suspended above simmering water. You can add different seasonings to the water to add flavour if you wish. Steaming is particularly good for cooking vegetables as it retains more nutrients than any other cooking technique.

Nowadays you can buy Chinese steamers with multi-level baskets which are ideal for cooking more than one food at once.

BOILING / POACHING
When boiling foods, especially vegetables, use only a minimum of water in the saucepan (except when cooking pasta), this way the nutrients in the food do not leach out into the water and lose you valuable nutrients such as vitamins.

Poaching involves gently simmering foods in water or flavourful liquids until cooked and is a great way to cook fish, and poultry. You will need a deep sided pan, deep enough to submerge the ingredients. The liquid should not boil.

BRAISING
Braising entails cooking food, meat, poultry, fish or vegetables slowly in a small amount of liquid at low heat in a tightly covered pot, usually in the oven.

The food is often quickly pan-seared on the hob to obtain colour before being braised in wine, stock or sauce. It is a great way to cook the tougher cuts of meat.

PAN-FRYING / STIR-FRYING
Pan-frying is a fast and efficient way to cook and seal in flavour but it is not the healthiest method as foods are fried in fat. However, using a non-stick pan will keep the amount of fat used down to a minimum as it requires little or no fat for the task.

When frying, I generally use olive, rapeseed or sunflower oil as they are high in unsaturated oils and low in saturated fat while also adding flavour. A non-stick cooking spray or oil-water spray is also suitable for the job.

Stir-frying became popular some years ago with our interest in oriental foods and cooking. It is quick, uses very little or no fat at all and preserves the freshness and colour of food, especially keeping vegetables crunchy and retaining the juices in meat and fish.

Stir-frying is a great way to get your recommended 5-a-day amount of vegetables.

Use a deep-sided non-stick wok or deep-sided non-stick frying pan.

MICROWAVE
Microwave cooking is a good low-fat method and particularly good for vegetables as it requires only a small amount of liquid for cooking, thus retaining all the nutrients as well as colour and texture.

PG tips

Here are a few do's and don'ts which you will find useful for eating more healthily and to help control your blood pressure by using little or no salt.

do's

● Avoid adding salt to your cooking and to your food at the table by enhancing the natural flavours of your dishes with herbs, spices such as onion, garlic (which may play a role in lowering blood pressure), lemon juice, flavoured vinegars, chillies, tomatoes and fruits. Use fresh herbs when possible at all times, dried herbs are fine but often have a 'grassy" taste when used in dishes and some herb mixes contain added salt (check the list of ingredients on the label).

● Use marinades as a way of adding flavour to your cooking. Marinating meat, fish and vegetables in ingredients such as low fat yoghurt, spices, herbs, lemon and lime juice, flavoured vinegars, all will add moisture, tenderise and aid flavour.

● When using reduced fat spreads for cooking, look for varieties that are over 40% in fat content.

● In dishes requiring the use of cream, use semi-skimmed low fat milks instead and thicken it in sauces with a little cornflour. In general use low or reduced fat products, such as milk, yoghurts and cheeses.

● Cook vegetables without adding salt and in a minimum of boiling water so that they retain their natural flavour and nutrients. Alternatively steam them with is a healthier option, as is roasting, baking and stir frying. Whichever method you employ, always serve them immediately once they are cooked.

● When using canned vegetables, pulses or fruits, always rinse them under cold running water to remove excess salt used in their making or, better still, buy products with no added salt which are often available in supermarkets.

● Use more vegetables and fruits which are rich in potassium such as asparagus, beetroot and bananas etc. Potassium rich food and drink is an important element in decreasing blood pressure, as it has the opposite effect in the body to sodium (the part of salt which can increase blood pressure).

● Feed your sweet tooth with natural sweetness with fruit, ideally use fresh fruits at all times, although canned and dried fruits are also good and still count towards your '5 A Day'.

● Do check labels on certain foods that you may at first think don't contain salt, such as breads or cereals, as many do contain a lot of salt. Always plump for wholegrain bread in preference to white bread which has more fibre.

● Always trim all visible fats from meats and skin from poultry.

● Many of your favourite recipes call for butter or oil. Using unsaturated oils such as olive, rapeseed or sunflower oil or a reduced fat spread instead lowers the amount of saturated fat in a particular dish. I do not generally use a lot of reduced fat spread in my recipes as I find it can noticeably change the taste of the food. The use of non stick cooking pans reduces the need for using lots of oil in cooking.

● Another successful medium for low fat cooking is the use of a oil-water based spray for pan frying, grilling or roasting. Simply mix together $2/3$ olive or rapeseed oil and $1/3$ water in a spray bottle. The oil mix can also enhanced by infusing the oil with herbs or spices for added flavour. There are also cooking sprays available commercially if preferred.

● In general look for ingredients and foods that contain little salt, but which provide your diet with plenty of vitamins, minerals and other nutrients.

● In the real world, it is not always possible to cook from scratch and there may be a need to buy pre-prepared foods. However, take the time to check food labels on foods which give healthier choices and are low in salt, saturated fat and added sugars, and high in fibre. For example, commercially made stock cubes can be rather salty in taste, so rather than using them, purchase a lower-salt packaged stock, available in sachet form from leading supermarkets and delis or, as a last resort, use half a stock cube to the same quantity of water.

don'ts

● Steer away from processed foods when possible, including fruits, fish, meat and vegetables that come ready-prepared in sauces. These often contain a lot of added salt, sugar and fats.

● By paying attention to the labels on food, you can reduce your salt intake dramatically.

● Once fresh vegetables have been prepared, never leave them uncovered and exposed to the air, or leave them soaking in water as their natural vitamins dissolve in the water and are lost.

● Try not to add sugar to fruits or salt to vegetables when you cook or serve them.

● There are numerous lower-sodium salt-alternatives on the market nowadays (which often contain potassium to make up the flavour). I personally find their taste unacceptable and advise you not to use them. In the long term, by far your healthiest option is to give up using salt completely in your cooking but you may find it difficult at first. I suggest you reduce your intake gradually as soon your taste will adapt and you won't miss it at all! The answer is to persevere.

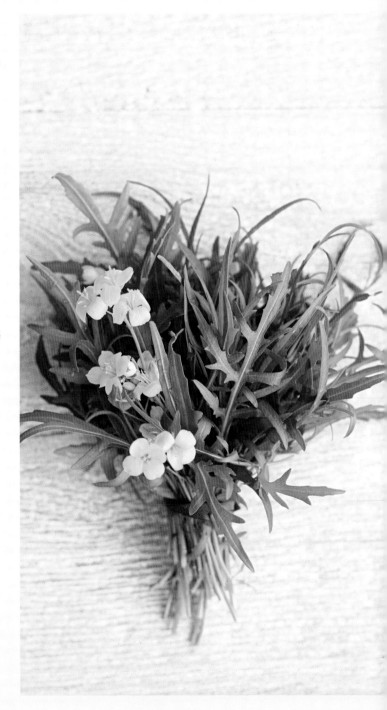

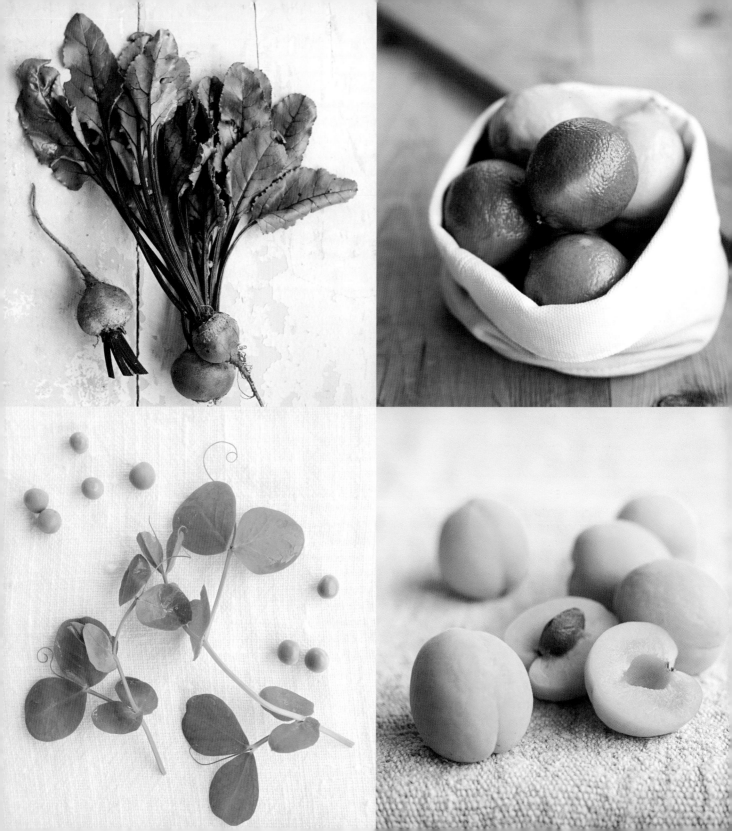

the healthy kitchen pantry

By using this list as a guideline you can create most of the recipes in this book and many more besides.

IN THE FRIDGE
Low-fat natural yogurt
Low-fat milk
Reduced-fat crème fraîche
Low- or reduced-fat cheese
Low- or reduced-fat salad dressing
Reduced-fat mayonnaise
Reduced-fat spread
Eggs
Fruit juices, freshly squeezed
Lean cuts of meat, fish and shellfish
Various freshly prepared low-salt stocks
  (ambient/sachet form)

FRUIT AND VEGETABLES
A wide variety of fruit and vegetables is essential for good health. Most fruit and vegetables are a good natural source of potassium and low in sodium, for example:

Asparagus
Beetroot
Carrots
Celery
Courgettes
Mushrooms
Peas

French beans
Potatoes
Tomatoes
Sweet corn, corn on the cob
Onions
Garlic
Squashes, various types
Fennel
Spinach
Leeks

Bananas
Apples
Pears
Lemons
Limes
Oranges
Pineapples
Blueberries
Nectarines
Peaches
Mangoes
Pomegranates
Melons
Watermelons
Figs
Soft red and black fruits
Rhubarb
Prunes

HERBS AND SPICES

Fresh herbs and spices are essential in low-fat cooking as they add colour and flavour to marinades that are excellent for replacing salt in recipes.

FRESH HERBS
Basil
Tarragon
Chives
Coriander
Mint
Thyme
Oregano
Sage
Flat-leaf parsley
Sorrel

Coriander (ground, seeds)
Cumin (ground, seeds)
Cardamom (ground, pods)
Cinnamon (ground, sticks)
Nutmeg
Chilli (powder, fresh, flakes)
Curry powder (try to find a brand with no added salt)
Black pepper (ground, whole)
Mustard (fresh, powder, seeds)
Saffron
Paprika (sweet, smoked)
Turmeric
Root ginger (fresh, ground)
Fennel seeds
Fresh lemongrass
Vanilla (pods, extract, essence)

CANNED AND PACKAGED PRODUCTS

When choosing canned and packaged products, look for brands with no added salt or sugar.

Oil-water spray
Cooking spray

Various flavoured low-salt stock cubes
Reduced-fat coconut milk
Tomato purée
Chopped canned tomatoes
Canned sweetcorn
Canned fruits, various types
Harissa
Couscous, various cereals
Dried beans, pulses
Dried fruits, various types
Fruit juices (cranberry, tomato, apple, peach nectar)
Olives in brine
Capers in brine
Wholemeal pastas
Rices
Flavoured vinegars (sherry, balsamic)
Olive, rapeseed, sunflower oil
Sesame oil
Vanilla pods
Various jams, reduced sugar
Reduced-salt soy sauce
Tahini
Honey, golden syrup, maple syrup
Wholemeal flour
Corn flour
Mango chutney

NUTS, SEEDS AND GRAINS
Hazelnuts
Almonds (flaked, ground)
Cashews
Pistachio nuts
Pumpkin seeds
Sesame seeds
Sunflower seeds

Wheatgerm
Coconut flakes
Rolled oats

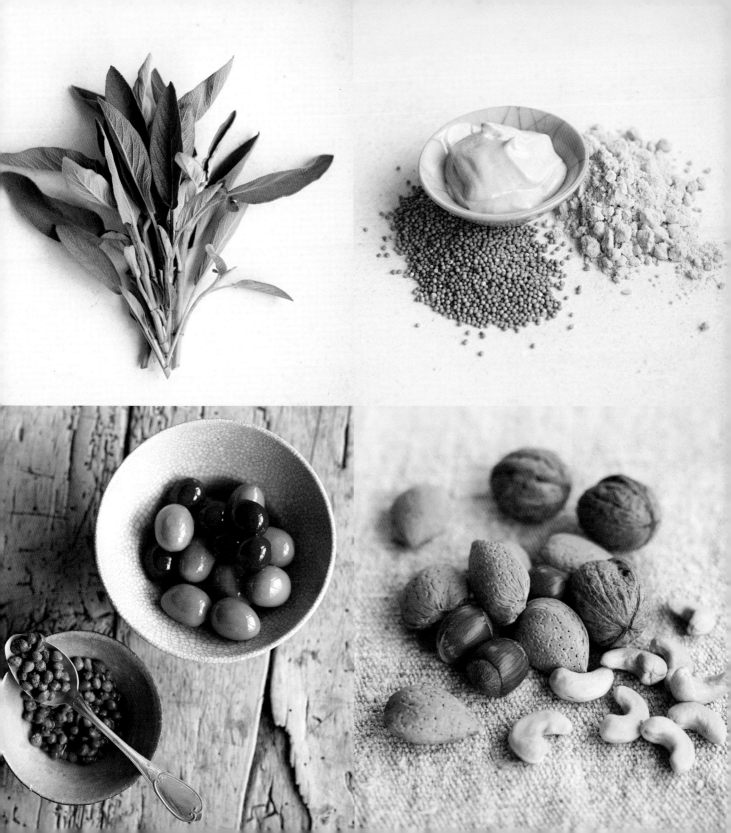

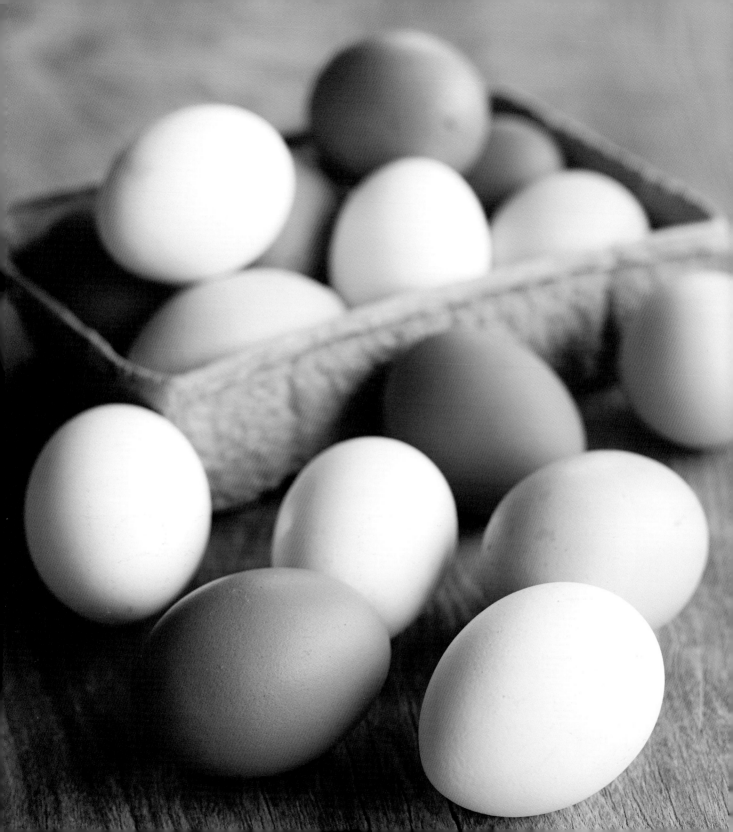

chapter one
breakfast & brunch

baked bean rarebit

For you baked bean lovers out there, and I know there are many, here is a great breakfast combo: baked beans on toast with a twist, topped with a cheesy rarebit crust on thick wholemeal toast – absolutely delicious.

400g dried haricot beans, soaked
   overnight, then drained
1 onion, finely chopped
1 tablespoon dark brown sugar
1 tablespoon black treacle
400g can chopped tomatoes
2 tablespoons tomato purée
1 garlic clove
1 tablespoon white wine vinegar

For the rarebit
45ml semi-skimmed milk
50g cheddar cheese, grated
1 teaspoon English mustard
1 large egg, beaten
pinch of paprika
4 thick slices wholemeal
   bread, toasted

Serves 4

Place the beans in a large pan, cover with 4 times their volume of cold water and boil for 10 minutes. Reduce the heat, partly cover the pan and simmer for 1–1½ hours or until the beans are tender (this can be done well in advance if preferred).

Preheat the oven to 170°C/325°F/gas mark 3. Place the beans in a suitable ovenproof casserole, add the remaining ingredients and mix together thoroughly. Cover with a lid, place in the oven and bake for 1 hour or until the beans form a thick sauce around them (add a little water while cooking if necessary).

For the rarebit, heat the milk, cheese and mustard together in a small pan over a low heat, until the cheese has melted. Add the beaten egg and stir until the mixture thickens, about 2 minutes. Do not overcook the egg or it will scramble. Season with the paprika.

Top each slice of toast with a pile of the beans, top with some of the rarebit and pop under the grill until golden. Sprinkle with black pepper and serve.

4 PORTIONS: 504 KCALS, 33G PROTEIN, 9G FAT, 3.7G SATURATED FAT, 78G CARBOHYDRATE, 15.5G SUGAR, 20.4G FIBRE, 0.86G SALT, 337MG SODIUM

grilled pink grapefruit with cinnamon

A simple but tasty breakfast recipe. The better the quality of your honey, the better it will taste. Look for a thick-set variety as runny honey tends to melt before it has time to caramelise. Pink grapefruit have more flavour and aroma than their yellow-skinned counterparts.

2 tablespoons thickset honey (alfalfa
   or clover for preference)
1 teaspoon ground cinnamon
2 large pink grapefruit

Serves 4

Heat the honey and cinnamon over a low heat for 5–8 minutes, then remove from the heat and leave to infuse for up to 2 hours.

Cut the grapefruit in half horizontally. Separate the segments from the membranes, using a grapefruit knife (or small knife), to cut around the outside. To help your grapefruit stand firmly, cut a thin slice of peel horizontally from the base of each half.

Heat the grill to the highest setting. Spread the cinnamon and honey mixture equally over the 4 grapefruit halves. When the grill is really hot, grill the grapefruit for 4–5 minutes – they should become lightly caramelised. Allow to cool slightly before serving.

4 PORTIONS: 54 KCALS, 0.9G PROTEIN, 0.1G FAT, 0G SATURATED FAT, 13.2G CARBOHYDRATE, 12.5G SUGAR, 1.3G FIBRE, 0.01G SALT, 4MG SODIUM

baked potato and porcini omelette

Porcini mushrooms are a gourmet-style mushroom, a real autumn treasure, not easily found unless you know where to find them and pick your own. Dried can be more readily available, but if not you can use thick slices of field mushrooms instead.

100g fresh porcini mushrooms (or 15g dried)
3 tablespoons olive oil
300g new potatoes, washed but not peeled, thinly sliced
1 small garlic clove, crushed
½ red chilli, deseeded and finely chopped
2 tablespoons chopped fresh flat-leaf parsley
4 free-range eggs
4 egg whites
freshly ground black pepper

Serves 4

Preheat the oven to 180°C/350°F/gas mark 4.

If using dried porcini, place them in a small bowl, cover with warm water and leave to soak for 45 minutes. Remove, drain well and dry them in a cloth. If using fresh, thinly slice.

Heat half the olive oil in a medium non-stick frying pan, add the potatoes and cook until golden and cooked through. Remove from the pan and set aside.

Add the mushrooms and remaining oil to the pan and fry until golden, then add the garlic and chilli and cook for a further 2 minutes. Return the potatoes to the pan, toss together with the mushrooms and parsley.

Take 4 individual mini frying pans or shallow ovenproof dishes and lightly brush with a little olive oil. Scatter the potato and mushroom mixture over the base of each dish.

Place the eggs and egg whites in a bowl, add a little black pepper and whisk until amalgamated. Divide the egg equally between the 4 dishes and bake for 40–45 minutes. Leave to cool for a minute before serving.

4 PORTIONS: 244 KCALS, 13G PROTEIN, 15G FAT, 3G SATURATED FAT, 14G CARBOHYDRATE, 1.2G SUGAR, 1.9G FIBRE, 0.43G SALT, 168MG SODIUM

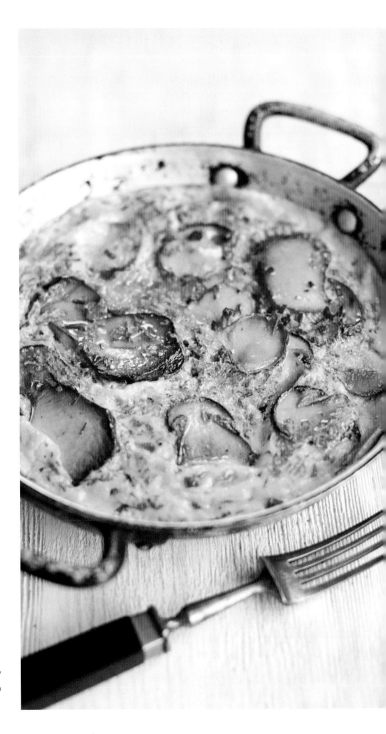

granola

This American-inspired breakfast cereal is becoming very popular here in Britain. You could add 100g raisins to the finished granola if you like, or try my summer-inspired version. Lovely served with fresh fruit and a good dollop of yogurt. This granola can be stored in an airtight container for up to a month.

75g flaked almonds
125g rolled oats
50g wheatgerm
60g sunflower seeds
60g sesame seeds
2 tablespoons sunflower oil
4 tablespoons honey or golden syrup
2 tablespoons brown sugar
1½ teaspoons vanilla extract
100g desiccated coconut or coconut flakes

Serves 8

Preheat the oven to 180°C/350°F/gas mark 4.

In a bowl, combine the oats, almonds, wheatgerm, sunflower seeds, sesame seeds and flaked almonds.

In a pan, heat the oil with 100ml warm water, add the honey, brown sugar and vanilla extract and almost bring to the boil. Pour over the ingredients in the bowl.

Stir the mixture well, then spread onto a large baking tray in a thin single layer. Place the tray in the oven and bake for 15 minutes, turning the mixture regularly to achieve even colouring. Add the coconut, mix well and cook for a further 15 minutes. Remove from the tray and leave to cool.

4 PORTIONS: 646 KCALS, 17G PROTEIN, 43G FAT, 10G SATURATED FAT, 51G CARBOHYDRATE, 24.2G SUGAR, 9.2G FIBRE, 0.05G SALT, 18MG SODIUM

summer granola

When the summer comes around my granola takes on a different guise, dusted with lavender sugar atop wonderful plump British berries.

To make lavender sugar, take 3 tablespoons caster sugar and mix with 1 teaspoon dried lavender flowers, place in a sealed jar and leave to infuse, ideally for up to 2 weeks, although it is fine to use immediately.

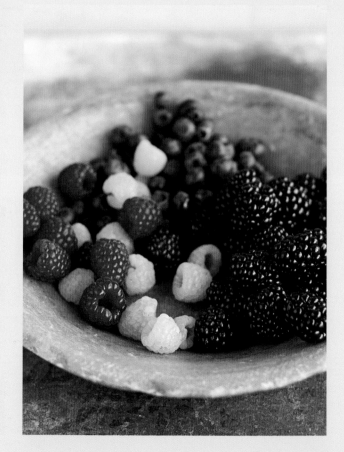

poppy seed pancakes with ginger fruits and mint syrup

Nowadays when we think of pancakes we often think of thick American style ones drizzled with maple syrup. Stop! Let's make way for thin French-style crêpes, which make an unusual breakfast. See my tips for making them in advance. This also makes a great late morning brunch. For the best results, leave the pancake batter to rest for 30 minutes before cooking; this allows the starch cells to expand, producing lighter pancakes.

For the batter
100g wholewheat flour
300ml semi-skimmed milk
1 egg yolk
1 egg
1 tablespoon sunflower oil,
  plus a little for frying
1 tablespoon poppy seeds

For the filling
2 tablespoons honey
juice of ½ lemon
1 cinnamon stick
300g mixed ready-to-eat dried fruits
  (e.g. apricots, figs, dates and sultanas)
2 tablespoons stem ginger in syrup,
  finely chopped
25g pine nuts, toasted
2 tablespoons chopped fresh mint
icing sugar, for dusting

Serves 4 (makes 12 pancakes)

For the batter, place the flour in a bowl, make a well in the centre, add the egg and egg yolk, the oil and a little of the milk. Whisk the flour into the liquid then gradually blend in the rest of the milk until the batter is smooth and free from lumps. Stir in the poppy seeds and leave covered for 30 minutes.

Cut the fruits into small 2cm cubes, place in a pan with the honey, lemon and cinnamon and cook over a medium heat for 10–12 minutes. Lift out the fruits and set aside, turn up the heat and boil the liquid for a further 5 minutes until syrupy in consistency.

Heat a little sunflower oil in an 18cm heavy-based crêpe pan or non-stick frying pan. Pour in enough batter (from a jug or use a ladle) to thinly cover the base of the pan, swirl the batter around the pan to thinly cover the base of the pan. Cook for 1 minute until small holes appear in the pancake. Use a palette knife (or for those a little more daring, flip it over) and cook for a further minute. Turn out onto a board.

Repeat this method until all the batter has been used (it should make about 12 pancakes). As you make the pancakes stack them on a plate, cover with foil and keep them warm under the grill or in a low oven. If you prefer to make your pancakes in advance, place the cooked pancakes on an upturned plate, cover them in clingfilm, and refrigerate ready for use.

To serve, spoon a little of the fruit mixture onto a quarter section of each pancake, fold in half then in half again, to create little pockets. Place on serving plates, drizzle over any excess mint-infused syrup, dust the plate with icing sugar and serve immediately.

4 PORTIONS: 514 KCALS, 11.9G PROTEIN, 21.3G FAT, 3.8G SATURATED FAT, 73.5G CARBOHYDRATE, 54.2G SUGAR, 4.5G FIBRE, 0.42G SALT, 167MG SODIUM

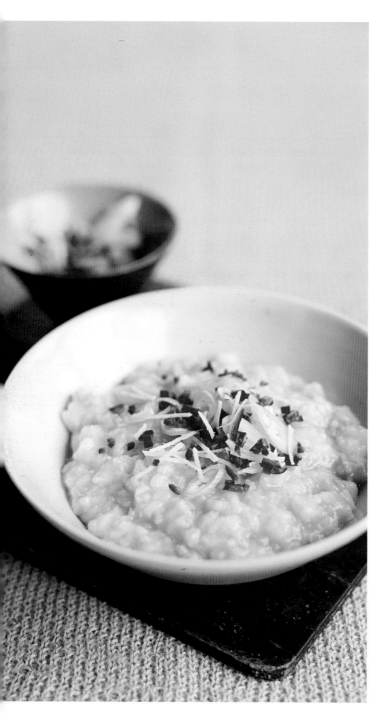

congee with spring onions and ginger

I have recently become interested in the origins of the Asian breakfast. At the Lanesborough we offer dim sum, scallion pancakes, steamed buns and rice porridge, known as congee. I prefer it simple and plain but often we serve it topped with chicken or fish. Congee is classically served with 'Yutao', a sort of fried bread doughnut that is available from Asian stores, but always serve with some chopped ginger and chopped red chilli, which is very popular in China.

200g jasmine or short-grain rice
1 garlic clove, crushed
2cm piece root ginger, peeled and finely chopped
2 tablespoons reduced-salt soy sauce
2 spring onions, thinly sliced

Serves 4–6

Bring 2 litres of water to the boil in a heavy-based saucepan. Add the rice, the garlic and half the ginger and bring to the boil.

Reduce the heat and simmer gently for 1 hour until the rice is well overcooked and almost puréed – it should be like porridge in consistency.

Add the remaining ginger and the soy sauce and stir through. Pour into 4 soup bowls, sprinkle over the spring onions and serve.

4 PORTIONS: 172 KCALS, 4G PROTEIN, 0G FAT, 0G SATURATED FAT, 41G CARBOHYDRATE, 0.9G SUGAR, 0.3G FIBRE, 0.9G SALT, 356MG SODIUM

jewelled porridge

As I have got older I find more often that I choose porridge as my preferred breakfast dish, especially on cold mornings. It is not only warming and filling, it is also simple to prepare. This recipe has a touch of the exotic about it, tempting, moreish and altogether beautiful to the eye. To remove the seeds from the pomegranate, remove them into a bowl of water, the seeds will sink and the white pulp membranes will float.

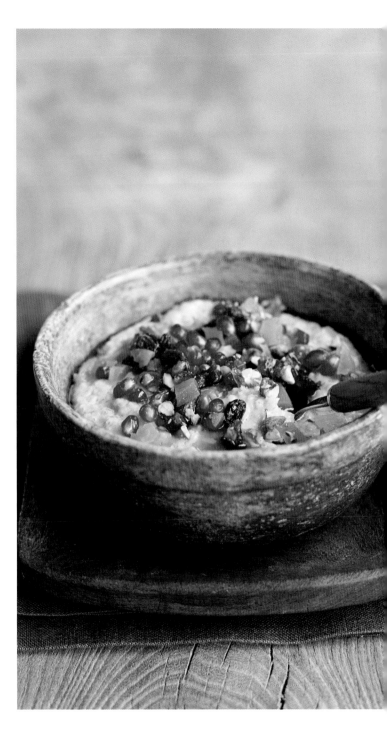

50g dried apricots (or canned), cut into small dice
30g raisins
25g dates, finely diced
2 tablespoons pistachio nuts (or flaked almonds)
1 fresh pomegranate, halved, seeds removed, drained and dried in a cloth (see above)
200g rolled oats
1 litre semi-skimmed milk
1 teaspoon orange flower water (optional)
3 tablespoons maple syrup or honey

Serves 6

In a bowl, soak the dried apricots (if using) and raisins in warm water for 1 hour until they swell in size. Drain.

Place the raisins, dates, apricots and pistachios and pomegranate in a bowl and toss together.

Place the oats and milk in a saucepan and bring to the boil, stirring constantly. Lower the heat, simmer for 3–4 minutes until thickened, and add the orange flower water if using.

Divide the porridge into 4 individual serving bowls and top each with a pile of the fruit mixture. Drizzle over a little maple syrup and serve.

6 PORTIONS: 296 KCALS, 11G PROTEIN, 8G FAT, 2.5G SATURATED FAT, 48G CARBOHYDRATE, 25.7G SUGAR, 4G FIBRE, 0.21G SALT, 84MG SODIUM

a few of my favourite wake-up shakes and juices

Sometimes I wake up and all I need is a refreshing breakfast juice or smoothie. At the hotel we prepare numerous, here are a few that get me motivated in the morning.

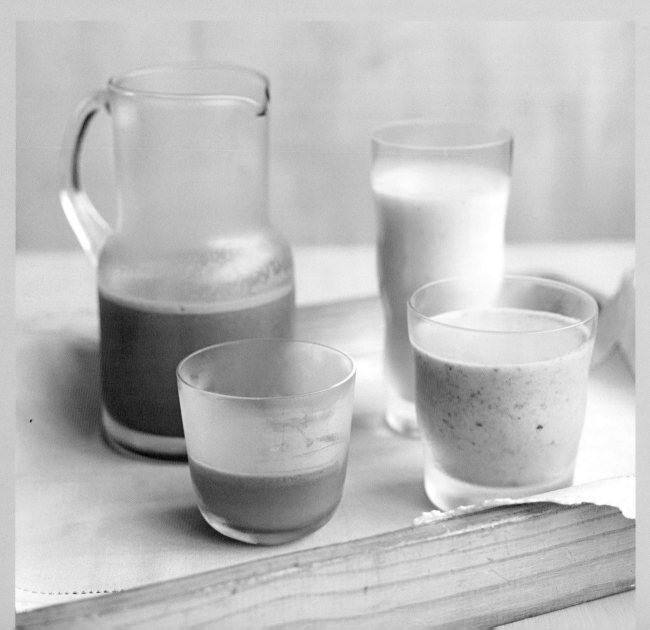

strawberry yogurt and passion fruit shake

4 small passion fruit, halved
100g fresh strawberries, cut into small pieces
225ml low-fat strawberry yogurt
1 tablespoon wheatgerm
300ml chilled semi-skimmed milk
honey, to taste

Serves 4

Scoop out the seeds and flesh of the passion fruit and place in a blender along with the strawberries. Add the yogurt, wheatgerm and milk and blitz until smooth and creamy in texture. Add the honey to taste, pour into chilled glasses and serve immediately.

4 PORTIONS: 109 KCALS, 6G PROTEIN, 2G FAT, 1G SATURATED FAT, 17G CARBOHYDRATE, 15.4G SUGAR, 1.4G FIBRE, 0.18G SALT, 72MG SODIUM

pineapple, coconut and banana lassi

1 medium pineapple
1 banana
150ml coconut milk
250ml semi-skimmed milk
juice of 1 lemon
pinch of ground cinnamon
honey, to taste

Serves 4

Remove the outer skin of both the pineapple and banana and cut into small pieces. Place in a blender with the coconut milk, lemon juice and cinnamon and blitz until smooth and creamy in texture. Add the honey to taste – this will vary depending on the sweetness of your pineapple.

Chill for 30 minutes in the fridge for best results, pour into glasses and serve.

4 PORTIONS: 190 KCALS, 3.6G PROTEIN, 5.5G FAT, 4G SATURATED FAT, 33.9G CARBOHYDRATE, 33G SUGAR, 2.8G FIBRE, 0.18G SALT, 73MG SODIUM

raspberry and orange smoothie

250g fresh raspberries
4 oranges, halved
sugar, to taste

Serves 4

Place the raspberries in a blender along with the freshly squeezed juice of the oranges and blitz until smooth and creamy. Add sugar to taste, again depending on the sweetness of your fruits. Transfer into chilled glasses and serve.

4 PORTIONS: 90 KCALS, 3G PROTEIN, 0G FAT, 0G SATURATED FAT, 20G CARBOHYDRATE, 20.4G SUGAR, 4.3G FIBRE, 0.03G SALT, 10MG SODIUM

watermelon and pomegranate juice

300g juicy ripe watermelon
250ml pomegranate juice, with no added sugar if possible
juice and zest of 2 limes
crushed ice

Serves 4

Remove the outer skin of the watermelon and cut the flesh into small pieces. Place in a blender with the pomegranate juice and lime juice and zest and blitz until smooth. Transfer to chilled serving glasses, add some crushed ice and serve.

4 PORTIONS: 52 KCALS, 0.6G PROTEIN, 0.2G FAT, 0G SATURATED FAT, 12.8G CARBOHYDRATE, 12.8G SUGAR, 0.1G FIBRE, 0.00G SALT, 2MG SODIUM

carrot, apple and ginger energiser

4 large carrots, peeled and cut into small chunks
4 Granny Smith apples, cored and cut into small chunks
2.5cm piece root ginger, peeled, finely grated

Serves 4

Pass through a juice extractor. Chill in the fridge for up to 30 minutes before serving to allow the flavours to infuse. Stir well together as it tends to separate, then divide between 4 chilled glasses, and serve.

4 PORTIONS: 143 KCALS, 2G PROTEIN, 1G FAT, 0G SATURATED FAT, 35G CARBOHYDRATE, 33.8G SUGAR, 6.6G FIBRE, 0.1G SALT, 39MG SODIUM

prune and orange compote with orange pekoe

Orange Pekoe is the term used to describe a medium grade black tea, normally associated with China and Sri Lanka. Orange Pekoe was once described by the Telegraph newspaper as the best tea to serve with a traditional English fry-up. I'm not surprised, here it forms a lovely syrup for a traditional prune compote.

300ml prune juice (no added sugar)
2 orange pekoe tea bags (or loose-leaf tea)
275g ready-to-eat prunes
2 juicy oranges
2 tablespoons chopped hazelnuts
low fat natural yogurt (optional)

Serves 4

Bring the prune juice to the boil in a small saucepan. Remove from the heat, add the pekoe tea and leave to infuse, uncovered, for 10 minutes.

Strain through a fine strainer into a bowl, add the prunes, cover with clingfilm and leave to steep overnight in the fridge.

Cut away the outer skin and pith from the oranges, then cut into slices over a bowl to catch the juices (ensure there are no pips in the oranges).

To serve, remove the prunes from the fridge, place in individual bowls and top with the orange slices. Add the reserved orange juice to the prune syrup and pour over the prunes and oranges. Scatter with hazelnuts and serve with a little yogurt if liked.

4 PORTIONS: 203 KCALS, 3.7G PROTEIN, 3.6G FAT, 0.2G SATURATED FAT, 41.4G CARBOHYDRATE, 41.3G SUGAR, 5.6G FIBRE, 0.05G SALT, 21MG SODIUM

banana-stuffed french toast

As a child I never remember having eaten French toast, not the sort of thing us East End lads ever wanted really. I often prepare it now for a weekend treat, usually strewn with all manner of colourful soft berries or stuffed with crushed ripe bananas.

4 slices thick-cut wholemeal bread, halved diagonally
1 large banana, ripe
2 eggs, beaten
½ teaspoon ground cinnamon
100ml semi-skimmed milk
1 tablespoon low-fat crème fraîche
1 tablespoon soft brown sugar
1 tablespoon grated orange zest
2 tablespoons icing sugar, plus extra for dusting
2 teaspoons sunflower oil
60ml warm maple syrup, to serve (optional)

Serves 4

Using a sharp knife, make an incision into the side of each cut slice of bread, being careful not to cut right through. Peel the banana and mash it in a bowl. Using a spoon, carefully fill each incision with the mashed banana and lightly press down to secure the filling.

Whisk the eggs, cinnamon, milk, crème fraîche, brown sugar, orange zest and icing sugar in a bowl.

Heat the oil in a non-stick frying pan over a moderate heat. Gently immerse each slice of banana-stuffed bread in the egg mix and fry for 2–3 minutes on each side until golden.

Transfer to serving plates, drizzle over the maple syrup if using to serve.

4 PORTIONS: 255 KCALS, 9G PROTEIN, 8G FAT, 2G SATURATED FAT, 40G CARBOHYDRATE, 21.7G SUGAR, 2.5G FIBRE, 0.4G SALT, 159MG SODIUM

portobello mushroom kedgeree

Portobello mushrooms are a fungi variety categorised as common mushrooms, like button mushrooms, crimini, etc. They are wonderful to eat, perfect for frying and grilling, and make a great breakfast mushroom with their meaty flavour.

2 tablespoons olive oil
8 large portobello mushrooms, thickly sliced
1 small onion, finely chopped
1 teaspoon mild curry powder
¼ teaspoon ground turmeric
4 cardamom pods, shelled, seeds removed
250g basmati (or brown basmati) rice,
   rinsed under cold running water for
   5 minutes, then drained
600–750ml hot vegetable stock (see page 156;
   if using ready-made stock or cubes use
   'low salt' varieties)
2 tablespoons roughly chopped coriander
2 hard-boiled eggs, peeled and quartered (optional)

Serves 4

Heat the oil in a heavy-based, deep-sided non-stick pan. When hot add the mushrooms and fry for 4–5 minutes until golden.

Add the onion, curry powder, turmeric and cardamom seeds and fry for a further 2–3 minutes to allow the spices to become fragrant.

Add the rice to the pan and mix well. Pour in the hot stock, stirring well, bring to the boil, cover with a lid and simmer over a low heat for 15–18 minutes or until the rice is tender and all the liquid has been absorbed.

Transfer to a large serving dish, scatter over the coriander and garnish with the hard-boiled eggs if using.

4 PORTIONS: 300KCALS, 9G PROTEIN, 7G FAT, 1G SATURATED FAT, 53G CARBOHYDRATE, 1.3G SUGAR, 3.5G FIBRE, 0.08G SALT, 31MG SODIUM

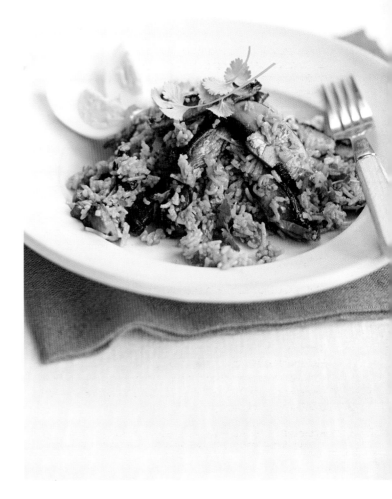

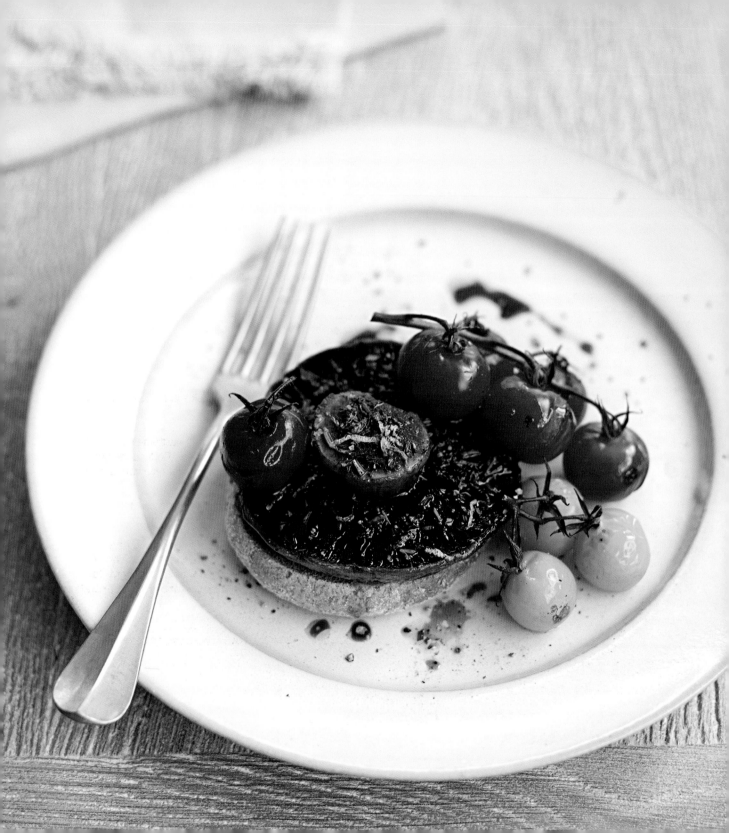

herb roasted vine tomatoes and mushrooms on toast

I often top these tomatoes and mushrooms with a poached egg, which when cut oozes over the herby tomatoes.

4 large portobello mushrooms, cleaned
2 tablespoons olive oil
1 teaspoon chopped fresh rosemary
1 teaspoon lemon thyme (or normal thyme)
½ teaspoon grated lemon zest
1 tablespoon balsamic vinegar
400g cherry tomatoes on the vine
4 wholemeal English muffins

Serves 4

Preheat the oven to 200°C/400°F/gas mark 6.

Place the mushrooms in on one side of a non-stick baking tin, drizzle over half the olive oil, then scatter over the herbs, lemon zest and balsamic vinegar. Roast for 10 minutes. Add the cherry tomatoes on the other side of the pan and roast for a further 5 minutes until all are softened.

Toast the muffins under a hot grill on both sides until golden. Top each muffin with a roasted mushroom and a cluster of the roasted cherry tomatoes.

Drizzle any resulting pan juices from the cooking over the tomatoes and serve.

4 PORTIONS: 243 KCALS, 10G PROTEIN, 8G FAT, 1.1G SATURATED FAT, 35G CARBOHYDRATE, 4.5G SUGAR, 2.1G FIBRE, 1.13G SALT, 444MG SODIUM

rhubarb and plum breakfast trifle

Seasonal fruits make for a wonderful breakfast treat at any time. This is my take on a simple breakfast trifle that's delicious and easy to make. Experiment with your favourite fruit combinations.

100g wheatgerm
150ml unsweetened apple juice
300g rhubarb, chopped into 2cm pieces
250g plums, stoned and cut into large chunks
1 tablespoon caster sugar
75ml low-fat natural yogurt, plus extra to serve
2 tablespoons flaked almonds, toasted
small mint leaves, to decorate

Serves 4

Place the wheatgerm and apple juice in a bowl, cover with clingfilm and refrigerate overnight.

Place the rhubarb and plums in a pan with the sugar and 75ml water, cover and bring to the boil. Reduce the heat to a simmer and cook for 4–5 minutes. Remove from the heat and set aside to cool.

Add the honey and yogurt to the soaked oats.

Divide half the oat mixture between 4 attractive trifle glasses, then top with half the rhubarb and plum compôte. Repeat with the remaining oat mixture and compote. Top with a spoonful of yogurt, scatter over the toasted almonds and decorate with mint, if using.

4 PORTIONS: 188 KCALS, 9.8G PROTEIN, 5.5G FAT, 0.3G SATURATED FAT, 26.5G CARBOHYDRATE, 19.1G SUGAR, 6.3G FIBRE, 0.05G SALT, 21MG SODIUM

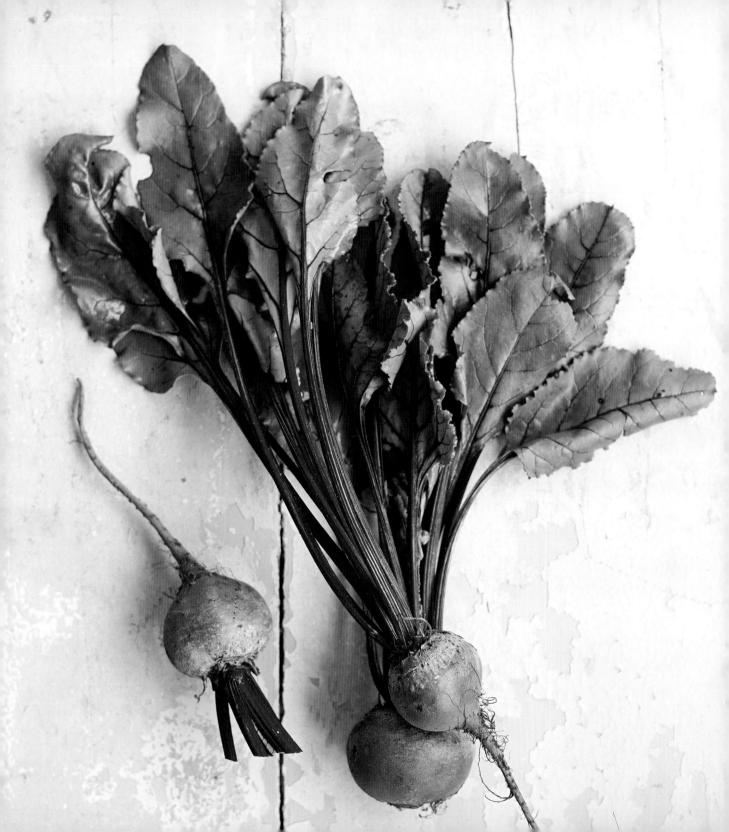

chapter two
soups & salads

avocado soup with three-onion salsa

A creamy, rich and velvety avocado soup, just the job to serve on a warm summer night. Look out for the Hass variety of avocado; it has a less waxy feel than the Feurte – you'll recognise it in the shop with its rough, dark green, almost purple skin.

2 large ripe Hass avocados
300ml cold vegetable stock (see page 156; if using ready-made products or stock cubes use 'low-salt' varieties)
300ml cold semi-skimmed milk
4 spring onions, chopped
juice of 2 limes
pinch of ground cumin
freshly ground black pepper

For the salsa
2 spring onions, finely chopped
1 tablespoon chopped chives
1 small shallot, finely chopped
juice of 1 lime
1 tablespoon maple syrup

Serves 4

Cut the avocados in half lengthways and remove the centre stones. Peel then place in a blender with the stock, milk, onions and lime juice. Blitz until smooth.

Season with ground cumin, black pepper and Tabasco, pour into a bowl, cover with cling film and refrigerate for 30 minutes before serving.

For the salsa, mix all the ingredients together in a bowl and season with little black pepper.

Divide the soup into 4 chilled soup bowls and top each with a pile of salsa in the centre.

4 PORTIONS: 262 KCALS, 5G PROTEIN, 23G FAT, 3.3G SATURATED FAT, 9G CARBOHYDRATE, 7G SUGAR, 4G FIBRE, 0.11G SALT, 45MG SODIUM

potato, wild garlic and sorrel soup

Wild garlic (*Allium ursinum*) grows in woodland near or among bluebells, and is readily identified by its garlic-like smell and long leaves. It grows from late winter but is at its best in spring. The flavour is similar to garlic, but slightly milder. It's also great in salads, especially towards the end of the season when they burst into bloom with tiny white flowers.

2 tablespoons rapeseed oil
2 small leeks, chopped
1 onion, chopped
200g wild garlic leaves, chopped
2 medium potatoes, peeled and cut into small pieces
50g sorrel leaves, torn into small pieces
1 litre vegetable stock (see page 156; if using ready-made stock or cubes use 'low salt' varieties)
150ml semi-skimmed milk
freshly ground black pepper

Serves 4

Heat the oil in a heavy-based saucepan, add the leeks, onions and chopped wild garlic and cook for 6–8 minutes until the vegetables soften.

Add the potatoes and stock and bring to the boil. Reduce the heat and simmer for 25–30 minutes until the potatoes are cooked.

Transfer to a blender and blitz until the soup is smooth. Return the soup to the heat and add the milk and sorrel. Stir until wilted, season with black pepper and serve.

4 PORTIONS: 147 KCALS, 6G PROTEIN, 7G FAT, 0.8G SATURATED FAT, 16G CARBOHYDRATE, 5.2G SUGAR, 3G FIBRE, 0.13G SALT, 52MG SODIUM

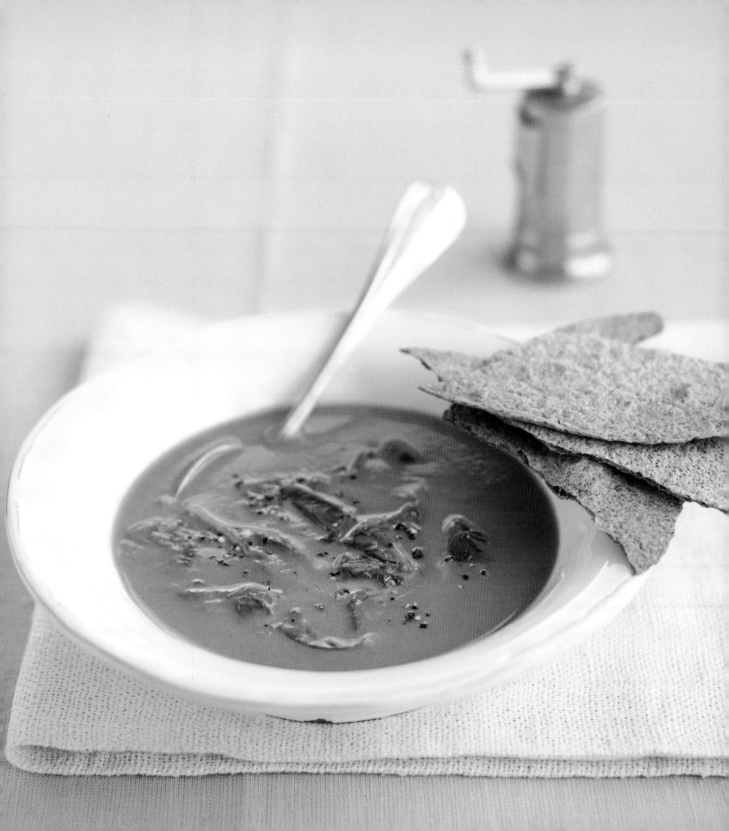

billy bi soup (spiced mussel soup)

This classic French soup made from mussels, saffron and curried spices is utterly delicious and very moreish. The majority of the mussels available in the UK are farmed rather than wild these days. Ensure that your mussels are plump in size and ensure that the shells are tightly closed when buying them. I recommend you eat mussels on the day of purchase.

750ml fish stock (see page 156; if using ready-made products or stock cubes use 'low-salt' varieties)
good pinch of saffron
1 tablespoon olive oil
1 small leek, finely chopped
1 garlic clove, crushed
1 teaspoon mild curry powder
60ml dry white wine
700g fresh mussels, cleaned
150ml semi-skimmed milk
2 teaspoons cornflour (mixed with 2 teaspoons cold water)
2 tablespoons chopped fresh chervil (or flat-leaf parsley)
freshly ground black pepper

Serves 4

In a pan, bring the stock and the saffron to the boil, then leave to infuse on the lowest heat setting for 8–10 minutes.

Heat the oil in a large saucepan, add the leek and garlic and cook for 2 minutes. Add the curry powder, cook for 1 minute, then add the white wine and boil rapidly for 2 minutes.

Throw in the mussels and pour over the hot saffron stock. Return to the boil, cover and simmer for 2–3 minutes until the mussels have opened.

Drain the mussels in a colander, then strain the stock into a clean pan. Remove the mussels from their shells, discarding any that remain closed.

Return the stock to the boil, add the milk, then stir in the cornflour mixture to thicken. Add the herbs and season with black pepper.

Divide the mussels between 4 soup bowls and pour over the hot soup.

4 PORTIONS: 111 KCALS, 9G PROTEIN, 5G FAT, 0.9G SATURATED FAT, 7G CARBOHYDRATE, 3.1G SUGAR, 0.9G FIBRE, 0.49G SALT, 195MG SODIUM

lentil, coconut and spinach soup

I love the earthiness of this soup. Any lentils could be used but I find the famous Puy lentils from France are as good as you can get and, for me, the best.

1 teaspoon cumin seeds
1 teaspoon cardamom seeds
1 tablespoon olive oil
1 onion, finely chopped
1 garlic clove, crushed
2 carrots, peeled and finely diced
175g Puy lentils
1 litre vegetable stock (see page 156; if using
 ready-made products or stock cubes
 use 'low-salt' varieties)
150ml reduced-fat coconut milk
handful of baby spinach leaves, stalks removed
freshly ground black pepper

Serves 4

Heat a dry non-stick frying pan. When hot, add the cumin and cardamom seeds and toast quickly for 30 seconds, moving them constantly in the pan.

Transfer to a mortar and pestle and grind to a fine powder. Alternatively, use a spice grinder.

Heat the oil in a pan, add the vegetables and cook over a low heat with the ground spices for 4–5 minutes until the vegetables are lightly softened. Add the lentils and stock, bring to the boil and simmer for 20 minutes until the lentils are tender. Add the coconut milk for the last 5 minutes of cooking.

Just before serving, stir in the baby spinach leaves. Season to taste with black pepper and serve.

4 PORTIONS: 234 KCALS, 13G PROTEIN, 8G FAT, 3.8G SATURATED FAT, 29G CARBOHYDRATE, 5.6G SUGAR, 5.5G FIBRE, 0.25G SALT, 99MG SODIUM

canteloupe melon soup with lemongrass and mint

This is an adaptation of a recipe from my first book, *Virtually Vegetarian*, a refreshing chilled soup that will rely on the quality of your ripe melon. If orange-fleshed canteloupe melons are not available, any type of melon can be substituted; watermelon makes a nice change.

1 ripe canteloupe melon
juice of 2 limes
2 tablespoons dry sherry
1 tablespoon balsamic vinegar
2 teaspoons caster sugar
4 sticks lemongrass, outer husks removed,
 inner part finely chopped
8 fresh mint leaves

Serves 4

Cut the melon in half and remove the seeds, then cut away the skin and cut into large chunks.

Place in a blender with the lime juice, sherry, vinegar, sugar and lemongrass, along with 150ml cold water. Blitz until smooth, then add half the mint leaves and blitz again. Strain through a sieve into a bowl and chill for at least 4 hours, the longer the better.

To serve, shred the remaining mint leaves and add to the soup. Serve chilled.

4 PORTIONS: 50 KCALS, 1G PROTEIN, 0G FAT, 0G SATURATED FAT, 11G CARBOHYDRATE, 9.8G SUGAR, 1.7G FIBRE, 0.04G SALT, 16MG SODIUM

spiced cashew nut and cauliflower soup

Cashew nuts are native to the north-east coast of Brazil, and have now spread to Vietnam, India and Africa. Like most nuts they are a source of fibre and protein and an excellent source of potassium, which can help lower blood pressure. However, due to their higher fat and calorie content, do not consume too many over a short period.

1 tablespoon olive oil
1 small onion, peeled and chopped
1 small cauliflower, cut into florets
1 medium potato, peeled and chopped
75g unsalted cashews
½ teaspoon ground cumin
pinch of ground turmeric
750ml vegetable stock (see page 156; if using
  ready-made products or stock cubes
  use 'low-salt' varieties)
150ml semi-skimmed milk
freshly ground black pepper

Serves 4

Heat the oil in a heavy-based saucepan, add the onions and cauliflower and cook for 6–8 minutes until vegetables have softened. Add the potatoes and cook for a further 5 minutes.

Add the cashew nuts, cumin, turmeric and stock, bring to the boil, reduce the heat and simmer for 15–20 minutes until the vegetables are tender.

Add the milk, then transfer to a blender and blitz until smooth and creamy in texture. Season with black pepper and serve.

4 PORTIONS: 224 KCALS, 11G PROTEIN, 14G FAT, 1.7G SATURATED FAT, 15G CARBOHYDRATE, 6.7G SUGAR, 3.4G FIBRE, 0.13G SALT, 52MG SODIUM

butterbean goulash soup

Although this soup is vegetarian-inspired, you can easily add 250g of lean minced beef to the vegetables, making it more hearty. I often like to serve this soup with some pieces of torn wholemeal bread toasted until golden in the oven or under the grill and drizzled with olive oil.

1 tablespoon olive oil
1 onion, peeled and chopped
2 carrots, peeled and cut into 5mm dice
2 sticks celery, peeled and thinly sliced
1 garlic clove, crushed
1 teaspoon caraway seeds, coarsely crushed
1 tablespoon Hungarian sweet paprika
1 x 200g can no-added-salt tomatoes
1 tablespoon no-added-salt tomato purée
good pinch of sugar
300g cooked butter beans
800ml vegetable stock (see page 156; if using
  ready-made products or stock cubes
  use 'low-salt' varieties')
2 tablespoons chopped fresh flat-leaf parsley
freshly ground black pepper

Serves 4

Heat the olive oil in a heavy-based saucepan. Add the onions, carrots, celery and garlic and caraway seeds and cook for 4–5 minutes until lightly softened but not coloured. Add the paprika and cook for a further 2 minutes.

Add the tomatoes, tomato purée and sugar, then add the butter beans. Pour on the stock, bring to the boil, reduce the heat and simmer for 20–25 minutes until the vegetables are tender. Add the chopped parsley, season to taste with black pepper and serve.

4 PORTIONS: 143 KCALS, 8G PROTEIN, 4G FAT, 0.4G SATURATED FAT, 20G CARBOHYDRATE, 7.9G SUGAR, 5.7G FIBRE, 0.26G SALT, 104MG SODIUM

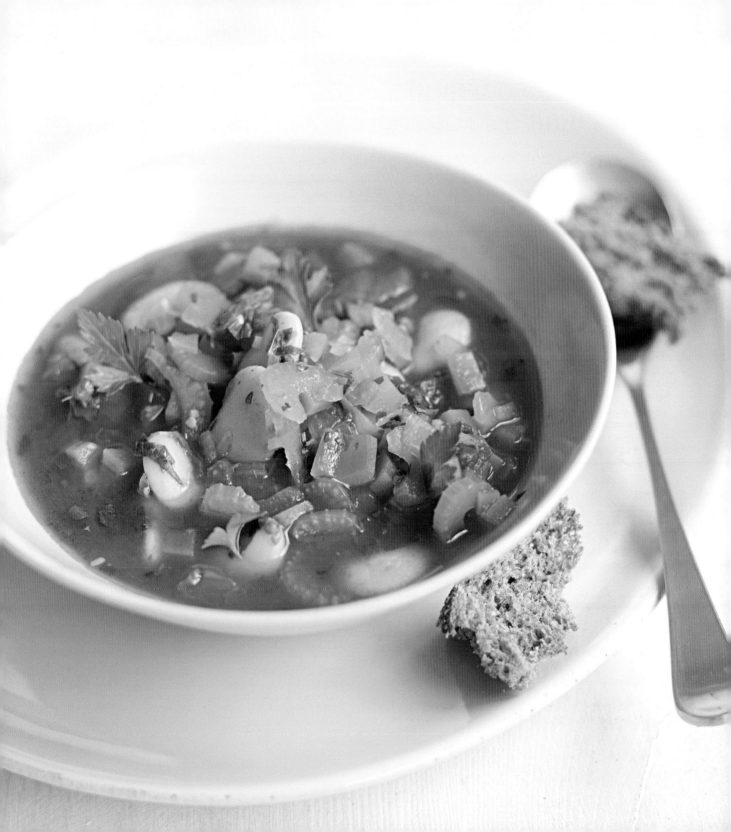

sweet potato, ginger and cinnamon soup

Sweet potatoes are very popular throughout America and many other parts of the world, but never really gained popularity in this country. This soup is a nice way to get your first taste if you haven't tried them before.

1 tablespoon olive oil
1 large onion, chopped
2 large orange-fleshed sweet potatoes (about 600g),
   peeled and diced
2.5cm piece root ginger, peeled and finely chopped
1 litre vegetable stock (see page 156; if using
   ready-made products or stock cubes
   use 'low-salt' varieties)
100g cooked brown rice
1 teaspoon ground cinnamon
1 tablespoon chopped chives
freshly ground black pepper
crispy wholemeal croutons (optional)

Serves 4

Heat the oil in a large saucepan, add the onion and cook gently for 5 minutes until it starts to soften.

Add the sweet potato, ginger and cinnamon and cook for a further 5 minutes. Add the stock and cooked rice. Bring to the boil. Simmer for 30 minutes until the vegetables are soft and tender.

Transfer to a blender and blitz until smooth. Serve hot with the chopped chives and some crispy wholemeal croutons.

4 PORTIONS: 221 KCALS, 4G PROTEIN, 4G FAT, 0.7G SATURATED FAT, 45G CARBOHYDRATE, 11.6G SUGAR, 4.5G FIBRE, 0.22G SALT, 88MG SODIUM

thai-style prawn broth

By using a good fresh fish stock you are guaranteed a lovely fragrant prawn soup, full of vitality and freshness.

1 litre fish stock (see page 156; if using
   ready-made products or stock cubes
   use 'low-salt' varieties)
5cm piece root ginger, peeled and thinly sliced
1 red chilli, very thinly sliced
2 sticks lemongrass, outer husks removed,
   inner finely chopped
4 lime leaves, finely shredded
50g baby spinach leaves
125g cooked rice noodles, broken into short lengths
4 spring onions, shredded
handful of fresh coriander leaves
225g sustainably-sourced cooked peeled prawns
freshly ground black pepper
juice of ½ lime

Serves 4

Bring the stock to the boil. Add the ginger, chilli, lemongrass and lime leaves, reduce the heat and simmer for 15 minutes.

Add the spinach, noodles and spring onions and simmer for a further 5 minutes.

Finally add the coriander and prawns, season with black pepper and add the juice of the half lime. Serve immediately.

4 PORTIONS: 175 KCALS, 16G PROTEIN, 1G FAT, 0.1G SATURATED FAT, 27G CARBOHYDRATE, 0.6G SUGAR, 0.4G FIBRE, 1.13G SALT, 443MG SODIUM

moroccan lamb broth (harira)

A classic Moroccan soup traditionally served to break the fast during Ramadan in many Middle Eastern countries. It can be a meal in itself, it is hearty and very tasty. Lemon is added at the end to give a characteristic tang to the soup.

225g lean diced leg of lamb, cut into 1cm cubes
1 tablespoon olive oil
¼ teaspoon turmeric
½ teaspoon ground cinnamon
½ teaspoon ground ginger
2 onions, chopped
2 tablespoons chopped fresh coriander
1 x 400g can no-added-salt chopped tomatoes
1 teaspoon harissa (or 1 small red chilli, de-seeded and finely chopped)
125g red lentils
125g cooked chickpeas (if canned, rinse under cold water)
50g vermicelli noodles, broken into 2.5cm lengths
1 egg, beaten with the juice of ¼ lemon
little extra lemon to serve (optional)

Serves 4

Place the lamb cubes in a saucepan, add the oil, spices, onion and coriander and stir over a low heat for 10 minutes, with no colour.

Add the tomatoes and their juice along with the harissa, then cover with 1.5 litres cold water. Bring to the boil, reduce the heat, add the lentils and simmer gently for 2 hours.

When ready to serve, add the cooked chickpeas and broken vermicelli and simmer for a further 5 minutes.

Stir in the egg and lemon mix with a wooden spoon to create egg strands. Season with black pepper and serve immediately with extra lemon, if liked.

4 PORTIONS: 392 KCALS, 31G PROTEIN, 13G FAT, 4.1G SATURATED FAT, 41G CARBOHYDRATE, 6.7G SUGAR, 4.7G FIBRE, 0.56G SALT, 220MG SODIUM

zaalouk (moroccan aubergines)

Zaalouk is a traditional Moroccan salad made of aubergine, tomato and courgette, cooked almost to a purée. It can be served hot or cold, eaten with a fork or as a dip. Traditionally it would be served with a Middle Eastern flatbread, but I also like to serve as a sort of Italian bruchetta on garlic-rubbed toast, which is equally delicious.

400g aubergines, cut into 2cm cubes
3 tablespoons olive oil
2 garlic cloves, crushed
1 red chilli, deseeded and finely chopped
1 large courgette, cut into 2cm cubes
¼ teaspoon ground turmeric
½ teaspoon ground cumin
½ teaspoon paprika
300g plum tomatoes, cut into 1cm cubes
3 tablespoons coarsely chopped fresh flat-leaf parsley
3 tablespoons coarsely chopped fresh coriander
freshly ground black pepper
juice of ¼ lemon

Serves 4

Bring a pan of water to the boil, add the aubergine and simmer for 15 minutes, then drain then well and dry in a cloth.

Heat the olive oil in a large non-stick frying pan, add the garlic, chilli and courgette and cook over a gentle heat until the courgettes have softened. Add the cooked aubergine and spices and cook for a further 5 minutes, then add the tomatoes. Continue to cook and mash the mixture with a spoon as it cooks to a coarse pulp.

When the mixture is well cooked, add the herbs, black pepper and lemon juice. Leave to cool – for best results, serve at room temperature.

4 PORTIONS: 122 KCALS, 3G PROTEIN, 9G FAT, 1.2G SATURATED FAT, 7G CARBOHYDRATE, 5.6G SUGAR, 3.5G FIBRE, 0.03G SALT, 13MG SODIUM

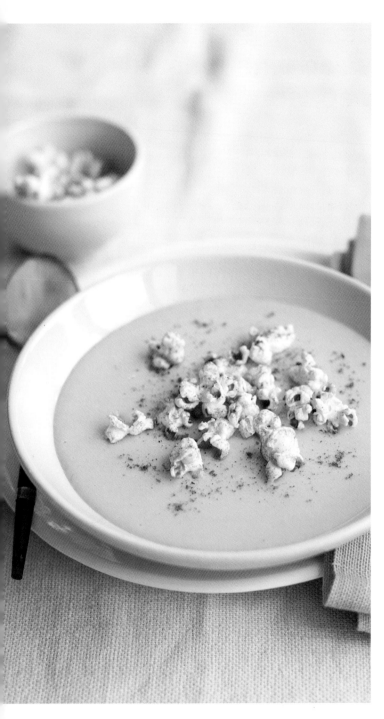

roasted sweetcorn soup with chilli popcorn

You will need fresh corn on the cob for this recipe – using the cobs helps to enhance the flavour of the base stock. Use unsalted popcorn.

2 large corn on the cob, in their husks
1 litre vegetable stock (see page 156; if using ready-made products or stock cubes use 'low-salt' varieties)
2 tablespoons olive oil
1 onion, peeled and chopped
white of 1 small leek, chopped
2 corn tortillas, cut into small pieces
150ml semi-skimmed milk

For the chilli popcorn
100g plain unsalted popcorn
pinch of chilli powder
pinch of ground cumin

Serves 4

Preheat the oven to 190°C/375°F/gas mark 5.

Place the corn in their husks ino a roasting tin, drizzle over 1 tablespoon of the olive oil and place in the oven for 30 minutes, turning regularly until charred all over but not burnt. Remove from the oven, peel of the outer husks, then scrape off the kernels with a knife and reserve.

Cut the cob into small pieces, place in a pot, cover with the stock and bring to the boil. Reduce the heat, simmer for 45 minutes, then strain, discarding the cobs.

Heat the remaining oil in a saucepan, add the onion and leek and cook over medium heat for 2–3 minutes. Add the chopped tortilla, stock and the corn kernels and bring to the boil. Simmer for 30 minutes. Transfer to a blender and blitz until smooth. Add the milk and season with black pepper. Keep hot.

For the popcorn, place in a bowl, add the chilli powder and cumin and toss well together. Serve the soup in hot bowls, topping each with a pile of chilli-flavoured popcorn.

4 PORTIONS: 402 KCALS, 10.2G PROTEIN, 20.4G FAT, 2.7G SATURATED FAT, 47.3G CARBOHYDRATE, 6.6G SUGAR, 2.9G FIBRE, 0.81G SALT, 321MG SODIUM

crab salad 'cocktail'

This dish is one of my favourite ways to enjoy fresh crab, bound in a fruity, low-fat crème fraîche with coriander and juicy citrus fruits. I like to serve it in a martini-style glass, which makes for an elegant presentation. Try to buy fresh crabmeat if you can.

350g fresh white crabmeat
juice of 2 limes
2 tablespoons maple syrup
1 teaspoon sherry vinegar
100g pineapple, cut into 1cm cubes
1 large orange
1 pink grapefruit
2 tablespoons chopped fresh coriander
  (plus extra to garnish)
2 tablespoons reduced-fat crème fraîche
50g golden raisins, soaked for 30 minutes
  in warm water, drained and dried
2 little gem lettuces, leaves seperated, and shredded

Serves 4

Take the orange and grapefruit and peel them carefully, removing all the pith. Using a sharp knife, cut between the membranes into neat segments, reserving the juices. Cut the segments into small dice.

Place the diced orange and grapefruit in a bowl and add the diced pineapple and raisins. Fold in the crabmeat and gently toss together.

In a separate bowl, whisk together the lime juice, maple syrup, vinegar and juices from the fruits. Add the crème fraîche and coriander, season with black pepper and mix well. Add the dressing to the fruit and crabmeat, season with black pepper and toss together to bind.

Arrange the shredded lettuce in the bases of 4 martini glasses, top with the crab mix, garnish with coriander and serve.

4 PORTIONS: 176 KCALS, 16G PROTEIN, 3G FAT, 0.9G SATURATED FAT, 23G CARBOHYDRATE, 22.8G SUGAR, 2G FIBRE, 0.95G SALT, 376MG SODIUM

cod and shellfish salad with roasted peppers

This makes a great first course or buffet salad. The seafood selection needs to be rinsed under a little cold running water to remove any excess salt.

150ml fish stock (see page 156; if using ready-made
  products or stock cubes use 'low-salt' varieties)
1 bay leaf
400g sustainably-sourced skinless cod fillets
200g roasted red peppers in oil, drained
2 garlic cloves, crushed
2 tablespoons roughly chopped fresh parsley
250g cooked seafood selection pack (prawns,
  mussels, squid), rinsed under cold water and dried
1 teaspoon sherry vinegar
juice of ½ lemon
3 tablespoons olive oil
freshly ground black pepper
pinch of smoked paprika
lemon wedges, to garnish

Serves 6

Heat the fish stock and bay leaf together in a small saucepan. Bring to the boil, then reduce the heat, add the cod and poach for 4–5 minutes until the fish is cooked and tender. Remove the fish from the liquid and set aside to cool.

Remove the bay leaf from the poaching liquid, return the liquid to the boil and reduce by half in volume. Transfer to a bowl and leave to go cold.

Cut the peppers into strips and place in a bowl with the garlic, parsley, seafood, chilled reduced stock, sherry vinegar, lemon juice and olive oil. Mix well.

Flake in the poached cod fillet and season with ground black pepper and smoked paprika. Toss lightly to combine. Serve garnished with lemon wedges.

4 PORTIONS: 328 KCALS, 34G PROTEIN, 17G FAT, 2.3G SATURATED FAT, 10G CARBOHYDRATE, 5.5G SUGAR, 4.4G FIBRE, 2.81G SALT, 1107MG SODIUM

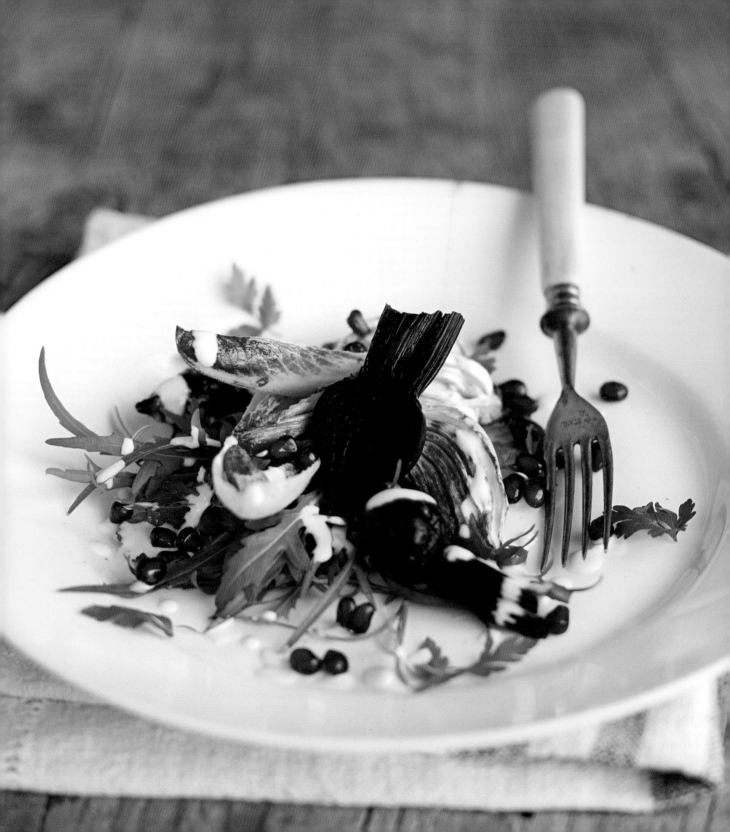

beetroot, fennel and pomegranate salad

If you do not want to roast your own beetroot, you can use ready-cooked ones (but not pickled!). To remove the pomegranate seeds, scoop them into a bowl of water: the seeds will sink and the white pulp membranes will float.

600g baby beetroot, with stalks attached if possible
2 tablespoons olive oil
2 heads of fennel, peeled and cut into wedges
2 heads Belgian endive (or chicory), leaves separated
250g rocket leaves
2 tablespoons fresh flat-leaf parsley, leaves only
1 medium pomegranate, seeds removed and drained (see above)

For the dressing
1 tablespoon tahini
100ml low-fat natural yogurt
1 teaspoon ground cumin
1 garlic clove, crushed
juice of 1 lemon
freshly ground black pepper

Serves 4

Preheat the oven to 180°C/350°F/gas mark 4.

For the dressing, mix the tahini, yogurt, cumin and garlic in a bowl, stir in the lemon juice and season with black pepper. Set aside.

Trim the beetroot, leaving some of the stalks attached. Place on a sheet of foil, drizzle over the olive oil, add the fennel wedges, then scrunch up the foil to secure the vegetables within. Place on a baking tray and roast for 1–1½ hours until tender. While warm, rub the skins off the beetroot and cut into small wedges.

Toss the endive, rocket and parsley leaves together and pile onto 4 serving plates. Top with the roasted beetroot and fennel, drizzle over the dressing, scatter over the pomegranate seeds and serve.

4 PORTIONS: 220 KCALS, 9G PROTEIN, 11G FAT, 1.6G SATURATED FAT, 22G CARBOHYDRATE, 18.1G SUGAR, 8.1G FIBRE, 0.35G SALT, 138MG SODIUM

roasted squash and coconut salad

The term summer and winter squashes can be confusing, as you tend to find one variety or another in the shops all year. Butternut and pumpkin are probably the most common squash varieties, but you can use most varieties for this salad.

1 small butternut squash, peeled, deseeded and cut into large chunks
1 onion squash, peeled, deseeded and cut into large chunks
2 large courgettes, thickly sliced
1 tablespoon olive oil
freshly ground black pepper

For the dressing
1 teaspoon red Thai curry paste
150ml reduced-fat coconut milk
juice of 2 limes
2.5cm piece root ginger, peeled and grated
2 tablespoons chopped fresh coriander
1 tablespoon chopped fresh mint

Serves 4

Preheat the oven to 200°C/400°F/gas mark 6.

Place the squash and courgettes in a roasting tin, drizzle over a little olive oil and season with black pepper. Place in the oven and roast for 25–30 minutes or until the squashes are tender and caramelised. Set aside to cool.

In a bowl, whisk together the ingredients for the dressing.

Place the caramelised squash in a bowl, pour over the dressing and toss together. Serve sprinkled with the peanuts.

4 PORTIONS: 194 KCALS, 7G PROTEIN, 11G FAT, 4.5G SATURATED FAT, 19G CARBOHYDRATE, 11.6G SUGAR, 4.9G FIBRE, 0.19G SALT, 76MG SODIUM

peppered tuna, watermelon and grapefruit salad

It is vitally important that the tuna is extremely fresh for this dish, as it is served only sealed on the exterior with the centre still semi-raw. The fruits work extremely well with the tuna, making a wonderful salad to grace any table.

4 x 150g very fresh sustainably sourced tuna fillets, cleaned of any blood and sinew
4 tablespoons olive oil
4 teaspoons black peppercorns, cracked
100g peeled watermelon, cut into cubes
1 avocado, halved, stoned and sliced
1 grapefruit, peeled and cut into segments (reserve the juices)
3 spring onions, finely shredded
1 red chilli, deseeded and finely chopped
juice of 1 lemon
250g continental salad leaves (to include watercress)
coriander cress (a new micro-green cress), to garnish (optional)

Serves 4

Preheat a chargrill or grill pan until almost smoking. Brush the tuna fillets with 1 tablespoon of the olive oil, then press each fillet into the cracked black peppercorns.

Place on the hot grill and cook for 30 seconds on each side to seal the exterior, then remove and set aside.

Place the watermelon, avocado, grapefruit segments and spring onions in a bowl, add the chilli, remaining oil and lemon juice and grapefruit juice. Toss together well, then add the salad leaves.

Cut each tuna fillet into 3 neat slices. Divide the salad between 4 serving plates, top with the peppered tuna, sprinkle over the coriander cress if using and serve.

4 PORTIONS: 413 KCALS, 38G PROTEIN, 25G FAT, 3.9G SATURATED FAT, 10G CARBOHYDRATE, 7.1G SUGAR, 2.5G FIBRE, 0.2G SALT, 79MG SODIUM

panzanella salad with grilled nectarines

Panzanella salad originates from Tuscany, and is often referred to as 'leftover salad', as it contains a vast array of ingredients in its make-up. Traditionally the bread is soaked in the dressing, but I like the texture of toasted. This recipe also includes grilled nectarines, which when in season give the salad a juicy freshness.

4 firm but ripe nectarines, each stoned and cut into 6 wedges
4 tablespoons olive oil
1 small white loaf, cut into 1cm cubes and toasted
300g cherry tomatoes, halved
1 red onion, thinly sliced
50g pitted green olives, rinsed under running water
1 x 125g reduced-fat mozzarella, cut into large cubes
300g rocket leaves
20 small basil leaves (or basil cress)
1 tablespoon white balsamic vinegar (or white wine vinegar)
1 garlic clove, crushed

Serves 4

Preheat a chargrill or grill pan until almost smoking. Brush the nectarine all over with 1 tablespoon of the olive oil, then place on the grill and cook for 4–5 minutes, turning regularly, until lightly charred all over. Remove, leave to cool and season with black pepper.

In a bowl, toss together the tomatoes, onion, green olives, mozzarella, rocket and basil.

Prepare a vinaigrette by whisking together the vinegar, remaining olive oil and garlic in a separate bowl. Season with black pepper. Add the vinaigrette to the tomatoes, toss together and add the toasted bread cubes. Leave to marinate for 20 minutes.

Divide the salad between 4 serving plates and top with the grilled nectarines.

4 PORTIONS: 485 KCALS, 21G PROTEIN, 27G FAT, 9.9G SATURATED FAT, 43G CARBOHYDRATE, 17.1G SUGAR, 5G FIBRE, 2.03G SALT, 798MG SODIUM

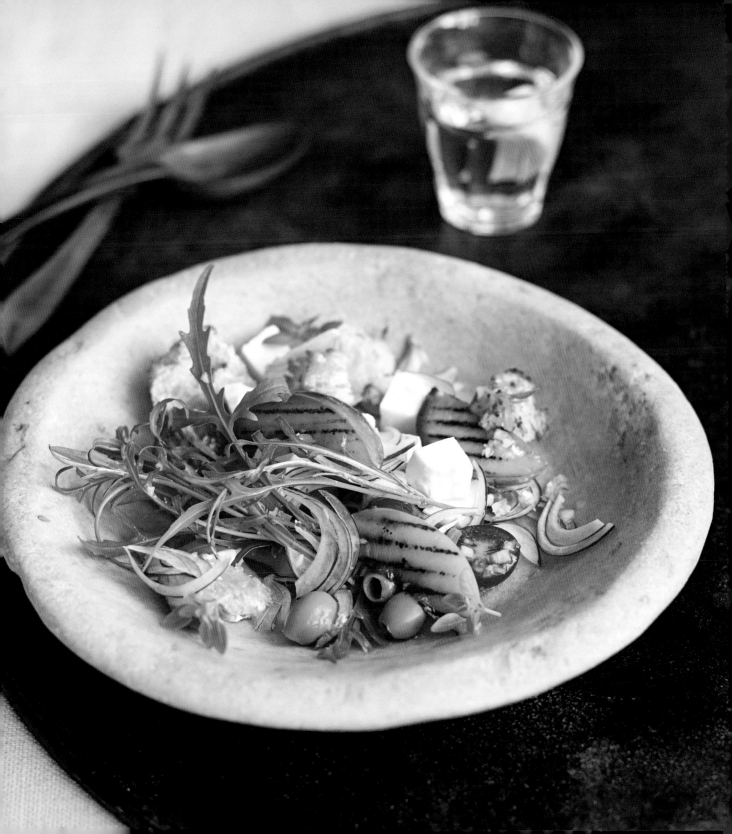

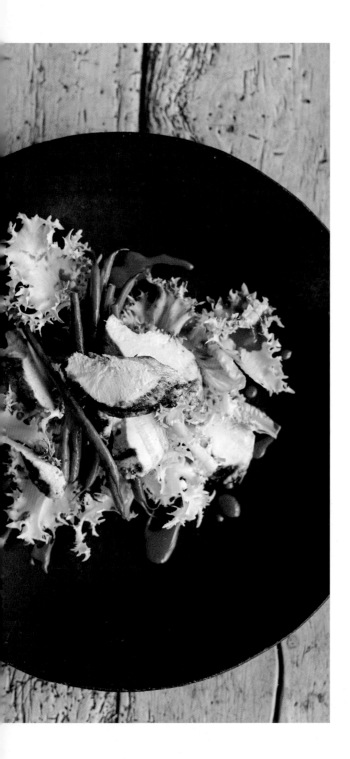

punjabi chicken salad

This Indian Punjabi spiced chicken salad is low fat, the beetroot-yogurt dressing is wonderful and if you love Asian food this salad is sure to inspire.

4 x 170g boneless and skinless
  chicken breasts
2 little gem lettuces
200g frisée lettuce
200g cooked French beans
2 tablespoons chopped mint

For the marinade
juice of 1 lemon
100ml low-fat natural yogurt
2 tablespoons chopped coriander
2.5cm root ginger, peeled

2 garlic cloves, crushed
1 tablespoon garam masala
½ teaspoon cayenne pepper
1 tablespoon sunflower oil

For the dressing
1 large raw beetroot, peeled
  and cut into large chunks
1 garlic clove, crushed
100ml low-fat natural yogurt
pinch of ground cumin
juice of ½ lemon

Serves 4

Place the chicken breasts in a non-corrosive dish.

Mix the marinade ingredients in a bowl and pour over the chicken. Cover with clingfilm and marinate in the fridge overnight.

Place the beetroot in a juice extractor, then place the juice in a small pan and reduce by half in volume until the juice becomes slightly syrupy in consistency. Remove to a bowl and leave to cool.

When cold, add the yogurt, lemon juice, cumin and garlic, season with black pepper and set aside.

Heat a chargrill or pan grill, when hot, remove the chicken from the marinade, brush with oil and cook for 6–8 minutes until golden and lightly charred all over.

Place the lettuces, French beans and mint in a bowl, add some beetroot dressing and toss together. Arrange on 4 serving plates. Slice the chargrilled chicken and pile onto the salad. Sprinkle with mint leaves and serve.

4 PORTIONS: 289 KCALS, 47G PROTEIN, 6G FAT, 1.3G SATURATED FAT, 11G CARBOHYDRATE, 8.2G SUGAR, 3.3G FIBRE, 0.53G SALT, 209MG SODIUM

lemon quinoa tabbouleh with grilled vegetables

Nutty-tasting quinoa (pronounced keen-wah) makes a nice alternative to the traditional cracked wheat in this recipe.

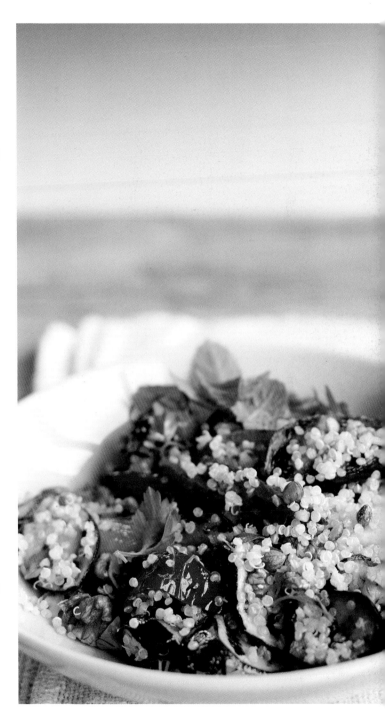

175g quinoa
450ml boiling water
zest and juice of 2 lemons
2 small aubergines, thickly sliced
2 courgettes, thickly sliced
1 red pepper, deseeded, quartered and cut into large cubes
1 yellow pepper, deseeded, quartered and cut into large cubes
1 head fennel, cut into 2cm thick slices

2 tablespoons olive oil
freshly ground black pepper
12 mint leaves, roughly chopped
2 tablespoons superfine capers, rinsed and dried
50g walnut halves, chopped
2 tablespoons roughly chopped fresh flat-leaf parsley

Serves 4

Place the quinoa in a pan, cover with the boiling water, cover, reduce the heat and cook for about 20 minutes until the grains are tender. Drain in a colander, transfer to a bowl and leave to cool.

Liberally brush the aubergines, courgettes, peppers and fennel with the olive and season with black pepper.

Preheat a chargrill or grill pan and, when very hot, add the vegetables and grill until cooked and lightly charred (you may need to do this in batches). When all the vegetables are cooked, add to the cooked quinoa.

Add the lemon juice and zest, capers, walnuts and chopped herbs to the quinoa. Mix together well, adjust seasoning and serve.

4 PORTIONS: 330 KCALS 12G PROTEIN, 17G FAT, 1.7G SATURATED FAT, 34G CARBOHYDRATE, 11.4G SUGAR, 5.5G FIBRE, 0.49G SALT, 191MG SODIUM

smoked chicken tortilla salad

This salad is a firm favourite ever since the day my good friend Dean Fearing, then the Chef of The Mansion on Turtle Creek in Texas, first prepared it for me. Here is my adaptation on the same idea.

1 carrot, peeled and finely shredded
1 red pepper, deseeded and finely shredded
1 green pepper, deseeded and finely shredded
1 yellow pepper, deseeded and finely shredded
2 tablespoons sunflower oil
2 corn tortillas
handful of fresh coriander leaves
225g sweetcorn kernels (canned without salt is fine, rinse under cold water and dry)
200g cooked black beans
400g sliced smoked chicken, cut into strips

For the dressing
handful of fresh coriander leaves
1 shallot, chopped
1 red chilli, deseeded and chopped
2 tablespoons honey
juice of 4 limes

Serves 4

For the dressing, place the coriander, shallot and red chilli in a blender with 100ml water and blitz a purée. Stir in the honey and lime juice.

Place the carrot and peppers in a bowl, add the dressing and toss well together. Set aside for 20 minutes for the vegetables to soften in the dressing.

Heat the oil in a non-stick frying pan, when hot add the corn tortillas and fry until crisp and golden all over about one minute on each side. Remove the tortillas and dry on kitchen paper, allow to cool.

Break up the tortillas into small pieces and quickly toss with the vegetables. Add the coriander, sweetcorn, black beans and chicken and toss again. Pile high on serving plates.

4 PORTIONS: 437 KCALS, 27G PROTEIN, 19G FAT, 4.5G SATURATED FAT, 43G CARBOHYDRATE, 14.7G SUGAR, 6.2G FIBRE, 3G SALT, 1182MG SODIUM

spanish roasted tomato salad

In this recipe oven roasted tomatoes are dressed in sherry vinegar, delicately seasoned with cumin and herbs. This salad is best made in the height of the summer when naturally sweet tomatoes and crisp broad beans are at their best.

12 medium ripe, firm plum tomatoes, cut in half lengthwise
1 garlic clove, crushed
2 teaspoons caster sugar
freshly ground black pepper
pinch of ground cumin
3 tablespoons olive oil
275g broad beans in their pods
2 tablespoons coarsely chopped fresh mint
4 spring onions, finely chopped
2 hard-boiled eggs, peeled and chopped

For the dressing
1 garlic clove, crushed
1 red chilli, deseeded and finely chopped
¼ teaspoon ground cumin
4 tablespoons olive oil
2 teaspoons sherry vinegar
¼ teaspoon Spanish paprika

Serves 4

Preheat the oven to 65°C/150°F/gas mark 3.

Place the tomatoes on a baking sheet, then sprinkle with garlic, sugar, black pepper and cumin. Drizzle over the olive oil. Place in the oven for 1 hour until the tomatoes have started to curl up at the edges and look shrivelled. Leave to cool. This can be done several hours ahead.

Pod the broad beans and cook in boiling water for 3 minutes, then drain and refresh under cold water. Dry in a cloth and remove the tough outer skins.

For the dressing, mix together the ingredients in a bowl. In a separate bowl, add the broad beans, mint and spring onions to the tomatoes, then add enough dressing to taste.

Place on a serving plates, sprinkle over the chopped egg and serve.

4 PORTIONS: 318 KCALS, 10G PROTEIN, 24G FAT, 3.7G SATURATED FAT, 16G CARBOHYDRATE, 11.2G SUGAR, 6.9G FIBRE, 0.17G SALT, 68MG SODIUM

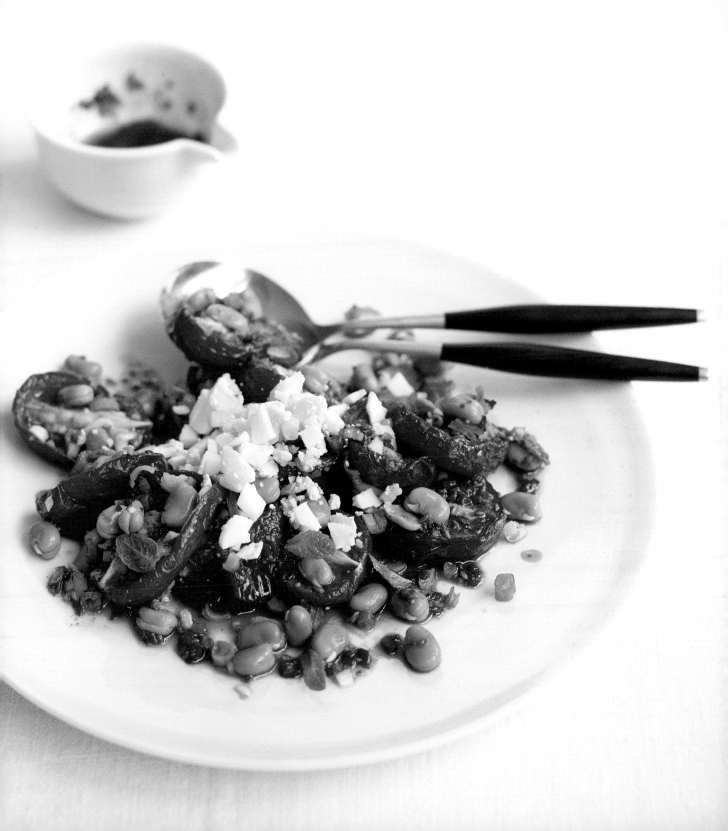

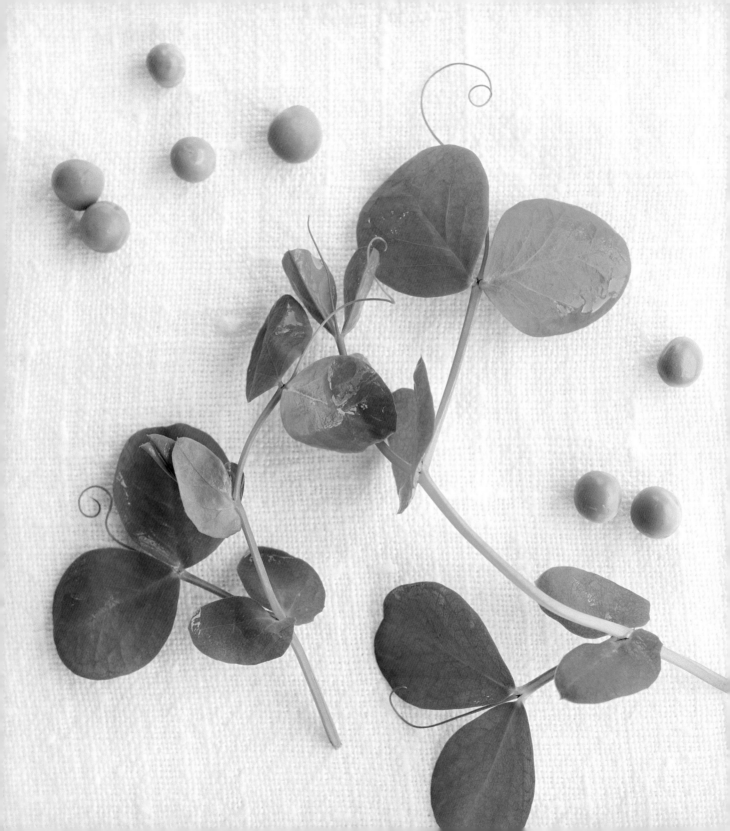

chapter three
starters & light dishes

crab cakes with prawns and harissa-mango salsa

Making cakes from pounded meat or seafood has been a tradition in many countries; they are easy to make and very tasty – and my recipe is no exception.

1 tablespoon sunflower oil
small micro cress leaves, to garnish (or watercress)
12 large cooked sustainably sourced large prawns,
   peeled and deveined

For the crab cakes
475g fresh white crabmeat
100ml wholemeal breadcrumbs
1 teaspoon ground cumin
¼ teaspoon ground turmeric
¼ teaspoon paprika
4 tablespoons reduced-fat mayonnaise
2 tablespoons chopped coriander
½ teaspoon dried chilli flakes
juice of ½ lemon

For the mango salsa
1 red pepper, deseeded and cut into small dice
1 small mango, peeled and cut into small dice
2 tablespoons chopped fresh coriander
2 tablespoons maple syrup
¼ teaspoon harissa, or 1 small red chilli,
   finely chopped
2.5cm piece root ginger, peeled and grated
juice of 2 limes

Serves 6

For the crab cakes, mix all the ingredients in a bowl. Season with black pepper and refrigerate for up to 4 hours to firm up the mix.

Divide the crab mix into 6 equal-size round patties, approximately 3 inches in diameter, and return to the fridge.

For the salsa, place all the ingredients in a bowl and season to taste with black pepper. Leave to infuse for 1 hour before serving.

To serve, heat the oil in a large non-stick frying pan, add the crab cakes, and fry for 3–4 minutes on each side.

Place the crab cakes on serving plates, top each with 2 prawns and spoon over some of the salsa. Garnish the top with micro cress and serve.

6 PORTIONS: 228 KCALS, 23.5G PROTEIN, 7G FAT, 1G SATURATED FAT, 18.9G CARBOHYDRATE, 10.9G SUGAR, 2.2G FIBRE, 1.76G SALT, 696MG SODIUM

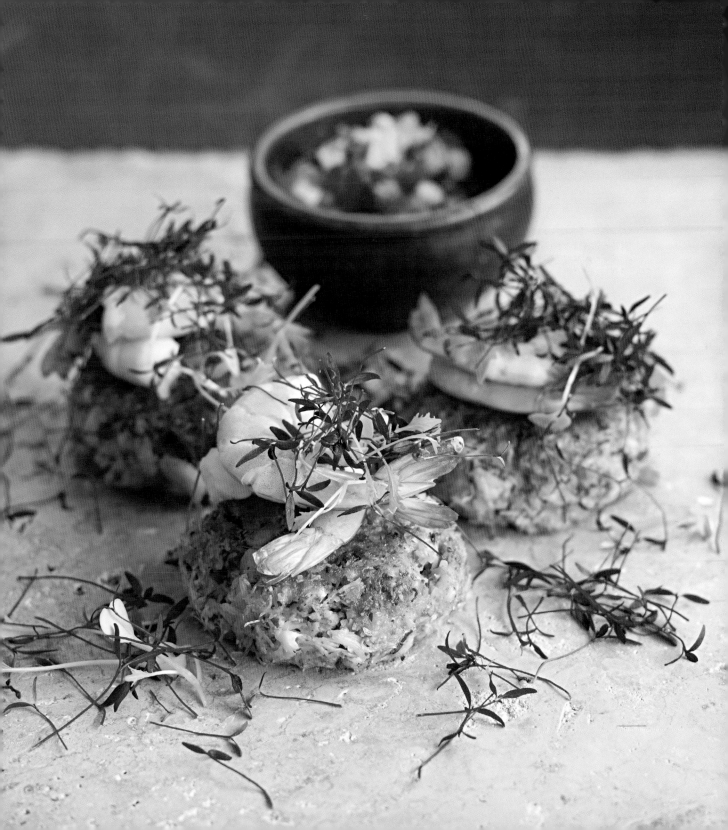

flat-leaf parsley risotto with lemon and prawns

The intense flavour of the parsley really works well with this risotto and the vibrant colour is visually amazing.

125g fresh flat-leaf parsley, washed
1 tablespoon olive oil
2 shallots, finely chopped
300g risotto rice (e.g. arborio or carnaroli)
1 litre vegetable stock (see page 156; if using ready-made products or stock cubes use 'low-salt' varieties)
425g sustainably-sourced raw tiger prawns, shelled, deveined and each cut into 3 pieces
zest and juice of ¼ lemon
2 tablespoons dry white wine
freshly ground black pepper

Serves 4

Plunge the parsley into a small pan of boiling water, blanch for 1 minute then drain. Place the parsley in a small blender with 100ml of the vegetable stock, blitz to a purée and set aside.

Heat the olive oil in a heavy-based saucepan, add the shallots, cover and cook over a low heat until softened. Add the rice and cook for 1 minute until the rice becomes translucent. Add the white wine and cook for 1 minute.

Meanwhile bring the remaining stock to the boil in a pan. Add a little of this stock to the rice and cook until the liquid has been absorbed before adding more. Continue this way until the rice has absorbed all the stock and is tender but still retaining a little bite (al dente).

Add the prawns, parsley purée, lemon zest and cook for 2 minutes. Season with black pepper. Divide between 4 bowls and serve.

4 PORTIONS: 377 KCALS, 27G PROTEIN, 5G FAT, 0.7G SATURATED FAT, 60G CARBOHYDRATE, 1.1G SUGAR, 2.8G FIBRE, 0.64G SALT, 254MG SODIUM

grilled sardines with thai relish

Fresh sardines are now more widely available. Here they are grilled in a Thai-spiced coating and served with a refreshing style relish.

12–16 fresh sardines, cleaned
2 garlic cloves, crushed
½ teaspoon dried red chilli flakes
2.5cm piece root ginger, grated
juice of 1 lime
2 tablespoons olive oil
pinch of sugar

For the relish
juice of 2 limes
75g unsalted roasted peanuts, chopped
1 red chilli, finely chopped
1 tablespoon sweet chilli sauce
2 tablespoons chopped fresh coriander
1 small red pepper, deseeded and finely chopped

Serves 4

Slash the flesh of the sardines 2–3 times on each side.

Mix the garlic, chilli flakes, ginger, lime juice, oil and sugar in a bowl, then rub the mixture all over the sardines to coat thoroughly. Set aside for 1 hour to infuse the flavours.

For the relish, mix all the ingredients together in a bowl.

Preheat the chargrill or grill pan until almost smoking. Place the sardines on the grill and cook for 2–3 minutes on each side until cooked through. Top with the relish and serve immediately.

4 PORTIONS: 442 KCALS, 37G PROTEIN, 29G FAT, 5.5G SATURATED FAT, 8G CARBOHYDRATE, 5.5G SUGAR, 1.5G FIBRE, 0.63G SALT, 247MG SODIUM

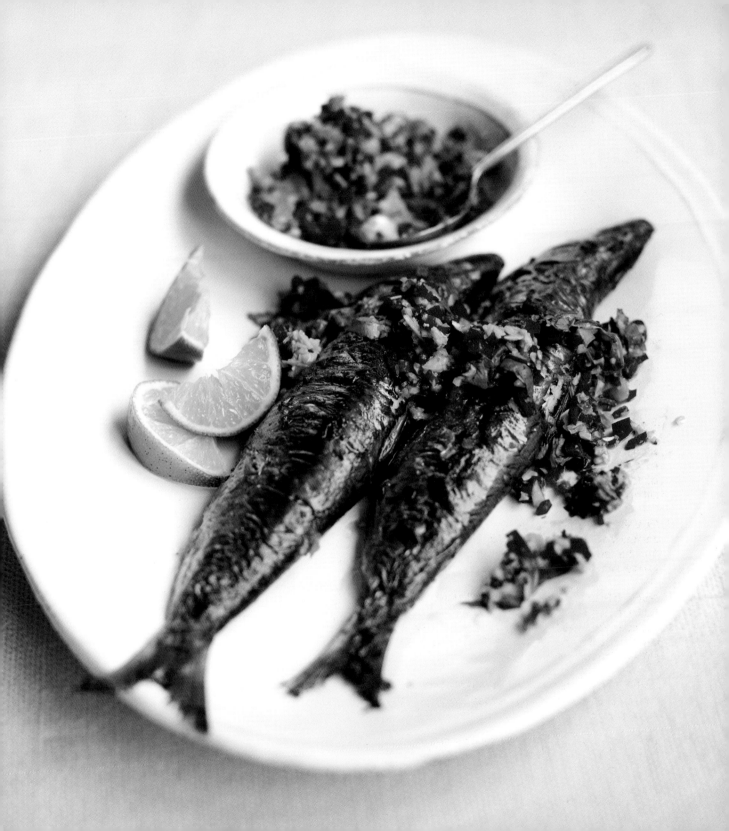

mackerel with haricot beans and horseradish aioli

It can be difficult to obtain fresh horseradish in many stores and supermarkets so I have plumped to use the creamy relish that is more readily available. However, these can be high in salt so check the label. You can prepare your own roasted red peppers if you prefer, but there are also some good jarred varieties now available.

1 teaspoon Dijon mustard
juice of ¼ lemon
3 tablespoons olive oil
450g cooked white haricot beans, hot
2 roasted red peppers, skinned and cut into small dice
1 red onion, thinly sliced
350g new potatoes, cooked, peeled and sliced
freshly ground black pepper
4 x 120g sustainably-sourced fresh mackerel fillets, boneless
good handful of rocket leaves
lemon wedges, to garnish

For the aioli
100ml reduced-fat mayonnaise
1 tablespoon creamed horseradish
1 garlic clove, crushed

Serves 4

Firstly prepare a lemon vinaigrette by whisking together the mustard, lemon juice and 2 tablespoons of the olive oil. Add the hot beans, roasted peppers, onion and potatoes and season with black pepper. Keep warm.

Heat a non-stick frying pan with the remaining olive oil, season the mackerel fillets with black pepper and cook, skin-side down for 2–3 minutes until the skin becomes crispy, then turn over and cook for a further 2 minutes.

Mix together the ingredients for the aioli and season with black pepper.

Arrange the rocket leaves on serving plates and top with the mackerel fillets. Place a little spoonful of aioli to one side and serve.

4 PORTIONS: 645 KCALS, 33.8G PROTEIN, 40.6G FAT, 6.7G SATURATED FAT, 38.6G CARBOHYDRATE, 8G SUGAR, 11.9G FIBRE, 2.12G SALT, 837MG SODIUM

marinaded salmon with pear and fennel

This recipe makes a wonderful starter for a special occasion. The fresh salmon fillets are cooked in a warm bath of olive oil infused with black pepper, star anise and fresh vanilla, which gives it a delicate flavour and an almost uncooked appearance.

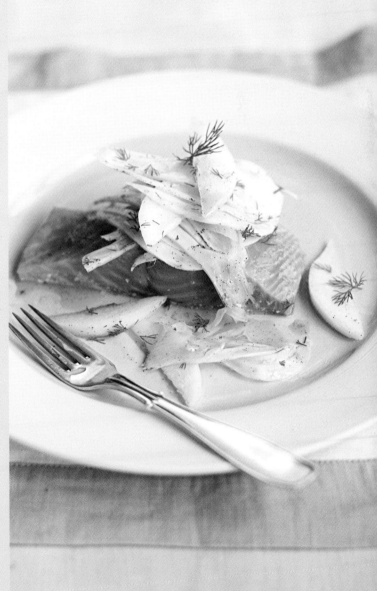

1 vanilla pod (or ½ teaspoon vanilla extract)
450ml mild olive oil
1 teaspoon cracked black peppercorns
3 star anise pods
4 x 150g very fresh sustainably sourced salmon fillets,
   skinless, boneless
1 large head fennel, fronds, removed, peeled and halved
juice of one lemon
2 tablespoons coarsely chopped dill
4 tablespoons olive oil
2 small firm but ripe pears, cored and cut in half

Serves 4

Take the vanilla pod and split it lengthways. Using a small knife, scrape out the inner black seeds into a bowl. Chop up the pod itself and place in a shallow saucepan with the olive oil. Add the peppercorns and star anise and bring the oil to a light simmer for 2 minutes, then remove from the heat and leave the flavours to infuse the oil. Strain the oil and return it back to the pan, using a thermometer heat it to 55°C.

Keeping the temperature constant, cook the salmon fillets for 12–15 minutes until cooked through (the appearance will be very opaque as it is cooked at such a low temperature). Transfer the salmon to a plate, pat dry with kitchen paper to absorb the excess oil and allow to cool.

Using a Japanese mandolin slicer, slice the fennel halves wafer thin, then add to the bowl with the vanilla seeds. Add the lemon juice, dill and olive oil. Slice the pears thinly too and add to the fennel. Season with black pepper and toss together.

Dress the salmon fillets on 4 individual serving plates, top with fennel and pear and garnish with more dill. Serve at room temperature.

4 PORTIONS: 633 KCALS, 31.3G PROTEIN, 53.4G FAT, 8.5G SATURATED FAT, 7.4G CARBOHYDRATE, 6.6G SUGAR, 2.7G FIBRE, 0.19G SALT, 77MG SODIUM

wholemeal spaghetti with sardines and raisins

In this recipe I have combined a Venetian speciality "Sarde in Saor" or soused sardines, mixed with spaghetti with added raisins to give a little sweetness. It works really well together.

12 fresh sardines, filleted and bones removed
a little wholemeal flour
2 tablespoons olive oil
1 small onion, thinly sliced
2 teaspoons caster sugar
60ml white wine vinegar
pinch of saffron powder
60ml dry white wine
450g wholemeal spaghetti
40g raisins, soaked in warm water for 30 minutes and drained
3 tablespoons pine nuts, lightly toasted

Serves 4

Lightly dredge the sardine fillets in a little wholemeal flour. Heat 1 tablespoon of the olive oil in a non-stick frying pan, add the sardine fillets and fry for 30 seconds on each side until golden. Remove and drain on kitchen paper.

Return the pan to the heat and add the remaining oil. Add the onion and sugar and fry for 5–6 minutes until golden. Pour over the vinegar, add the saffron and white wine and cook for 2–3 minutes. Remove from the pan and set aside.

Lay the sardine fillets in a dish, layered with the onions. Leave for 2 hours before use.

Cook the spaghetti in a large pan of boiling water until al dente, then drain in a colander. Return to the pan, add the sardines and onion, then the raisins and pine nuts. Toss together, season with black pepper and serve.

4 PORTIONS: 795 KCALS, 51G PROTEIN, 29G FAT, 4.9G SATURATED FAT, 87G CARBOHYDRATE, 15.2G SUGAR, 10.2G FIBRE, 0.9G SALT, 355MG SODIUM

mussel bouillabaise

I adore mussels prepared any style, but this one is very French in its make-up. The sauce has a warming glow about it and an aniseed flavour. Top with the garlic toasted slices of French bread.

1 tablespoon olive oil
1 onion, finely chopped
1 garlic clove, crushed
1 small bulb fennel, peeled and finely chopped
400g can chopped tomatoes (no added salt)
½ teaspoon thyme leaves
1 small bay leaf
juice and zest of ½ orange
700ml fish stock (see page 156; if using ready-made stock or cubes use 'low salt' varieties)
pinch of saffron
3 tablespoons Pernod
1 kg cleaned mussels
1 tablespoon chopped fresh flat-leaf parsley
4 slices baguette, toasted and rubbed with garlic and olive oil (optional)

Serves 4

Heat the olive oil in a large saucepan. Add the onion, garlic and fennel and cook for 10–12 minutes until the vegetables are soft and just starting to colour.

Add the tomatoes, thyme, bay leaf, orange zest and juice and cook for 5 minutes.

Pour in the fish stock, saffron and Pernod and bring to the boil. Throw in the cleaned mussels, cover with a lid and cook for 3–4 minutes until the mussels have opened. Discard any that remain closed. Transfer to serving dishes, pour over the cooking sauce, sprinkle over the chopped parsley and serve with the toasted baguette.

4 PORTIONS: 199 KCALS, 14G PROTEIN, 5G FAT, 0.7G SATURATED FAT, 20G CARBOHYDRATE, 5.9G SUGAR, 2.9G FIBRE, 1.05G SALT, 414MG SODIUM

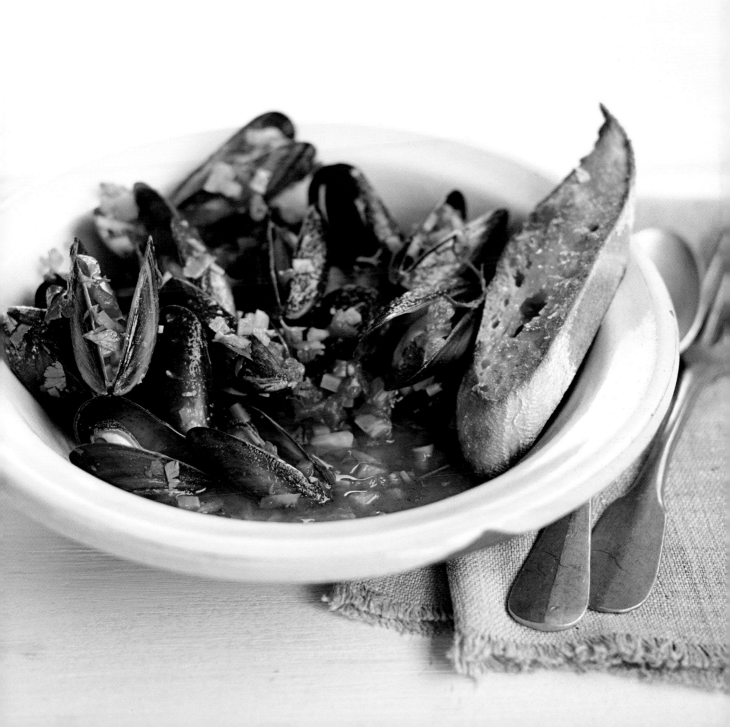

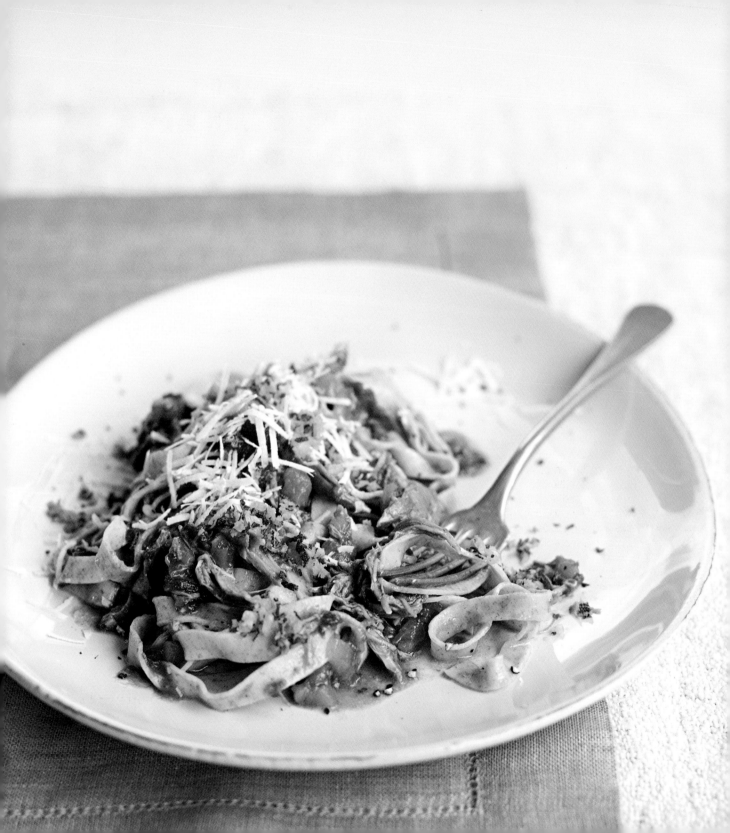

pasta with duck ragu, orange and sage gremolata

With its rustic texture, wholemeal pasta stands up well to bold, earthy sauces.

450g dried wholemeal noodles (tagliatelle or penne)

For the duck ragu
3 tablespoons olive oil
4 fresh duck legs, skin removed
freshly ground black pepper
1 onion, peeled and chopped
1 carrot, peeled and chopped
2 garlic cloves, crushed
4 sage leaves, chopped
100ml red wine

300ml chicken stock (see page 156; if using ready made stock or cubes use 'low salt' varieties)
200g can chopped tomatoes
2 tablespoons freshly grated parmesan

For the gremolata
4 sage leaves, finely chopped
zest of 1 orange
½ garlic clove, crushed
2 tablespoons olive oil

Serves 6

First make the duck ragu. Heat the oil in a heavy-based flameproof casserole or pan. Season the duck legs with black pepper and add to the pan, turning them until coloured all over. Transfer to a plate. Add the onions, carrot and garlic to the pan juices and fry until lightly golden. Add the wine, stock tomatoes and bring to the boil. Add the sage and reduce to a simmer. Cover with a lid and simmer for 1 hour.

Transfer the duck to a plate and allow to cool, remove the meat from the bones, then return the meat to the sauce, cook for a further 10 minutes. Season and keep warm.

For the gremolata, toss all the ingredients together in a bowl. Cook the pasta in boiling water until just al dente, then drain in a colander.

To serve, stir the duck ragu sauce into the pasta, then divide between 4 serving bowls. Sprinkle over a little parmesan, then the orange-sage gremolata.and grill for 3–4 minutes on each side until cooked and lightly charred all over.

4 PORTIONS: 242 KCALS, 20G PROTEIN, 17G FAT, 2.8G SATURATED FAT, 4G CARBOHYDRATE, 1.2G SUGAR, 0.1G FIBRE, 1.07G SALT, 422MG SODIUM

tunisian chicken liver kebabs with lemon mayonnaise

If you're a lover of offal like me you'll love these easily prepared chicken livers. Great cooked on a barbecue.

20 fresh (or frozen) chicken livers (about 450g), any green bile removed
1 tablespoon olive oil
1 teaspoon ground cumin
1 teaspoon smoked paprika
2 tablespoons white wine vinegar
freshly ground black pepper

For the lemon mayonnaise
150ml reduced-fat mayonnaise
zest and juice of 1 lemon
2 spring onions, very finely chopped
1 tablespoon chopped fresh coriander

Serves 4

Dry the chicken livers with kitchen paper to remove excess moisture. In a bowl combine the oil, spices and vinegar. Add the chicken livers and leave to marinate for 1 hour. Soak 4 wooden skewers in water.

Carefully thread 5 chicken livers onto each skewer. Brush with the marinade.

Heat a chargrill or pan grill until very hot, add the skewers and grill for 3–4 minutes on each side until cooked and lightly charred all over.

Mix the ingredients for the lemon mayonnaise in a bowl and season with black pepper.

Serve the kebabs and mayonnaise with a crisp green salad and warm pitta bread fingers.

4 PORTIONS: 242 KCALS, 20G PROTEIN, 17G FAT, 2.8G SATURATED FAT, 4G CARBOHYDRATE, 1.2G SUGAR, 0.1G FIBRE, 1.07G SALT, 422MG SODIUM

portobello mushrooms al forno

'Al forno' is an Italian culinary term describing food that is baked or passed through an oven.

8 large portobello mushrooms, stalks
  removed and reserved
2 teaspoons olive oil
1 onion, finely chopped
200g cooked spinach leaves, chopped
75g sun-dried tomatoes (not in oil), chopped
175g reduced-fat mozzarella, cut into small cubes
1 egg yolk
freshly ground black pepper
50g wholemeal breadcrumbs
2 tablespoons prepared pesto

Serves 4

Preheat oven to 200°C/400°F/gas mark 6.

Chop the mushroom stalks finely. Heat half the olive oil in a non-stick pan, add the onion and chopped mushroom stalks and cook over a low heat until softened.

Add the spinach and tomatoes and mix well. Transfer to a bowl and set aside until cold.

Add the mozzarella, mix well, then stir in the egg yolk. Season with black pepper.

Brush the mushroom cups liberally with the remaining olive oil, then fill each with the filling. Place the stuffed mushrooms in a single layer in an ovenproof dish.

In a bowl, mix the breadcrumbs, the remaining olive oil and the pesto, then sprinkle liberally over the mushrooms. Bake for 8–10 minutes until tender with a lightly golden crust.

4 PORTIONS: 236 KCALS, 18.3G PROTEIN, 12.1G FAT, 4.4G SATURATED FAT, 14.3G CARBOHYDRATE, 5.1G SUGAR, 4.3G FIBRE, 0.94G SALT, 370MG SODIUM

goan egg, tofu and chickpea curry

Being a great lover of eggs, I adore this curry made with eggs, chickpeas and firm tofu; it makes a lovely vegetarian dish. Serve with steamed basmati rice. Tamarind paste often contains salt, so check the label.

6 freshly cooked hard-boiled eggs
  (I recommend 8 minutes), peeled
1 onion, thinly sliced
½ teaspoon red chilli powder
¼ teaspoon ground turmeric
1 teaspoon ground coriander
¼ teaspoon ground cumin
1 tablespoon tamarind paste
2 good handfuls of young baby spinach,
  stalks removed
4 plum tomatoes, cut into 1cm cubes
1 x 400ml can reduced-fat coconut milk
1 tablespoon sunflower oil
300g firm tofu, cut into 1cm cubes
150g cooked chickpeas
2 tablespoons chopped fresh coriander

Serves 4

Heat the oil in a saucepan, add the onions and cook for 5 minutes until softened. Add the tofu and cook for 2 minutes. Add the spices and cook over a gentle heat for a further 5 minutes.

Add the baby spinach and coriander and cook until it wilts down, about 2 minutes. Add the tomatoes, coconut milk and tamarind paste, simmer gently for a further 5 minutes.

Cut the hard-boiled eggs in half and add to the curry along with the chickpeas. Season with black pepper and gently heat through. Serve with the steamed rice.

4 PORTIONS: 385 KCALS, 21.7G PROTEIN, 26.0G FAT, 12.4G SATURATED FAT, 17.9G CARBOHYDRATE, 8.5G SUGAR, 4.1G FIBRE, 0.82G SALT, 325MG SODIUM

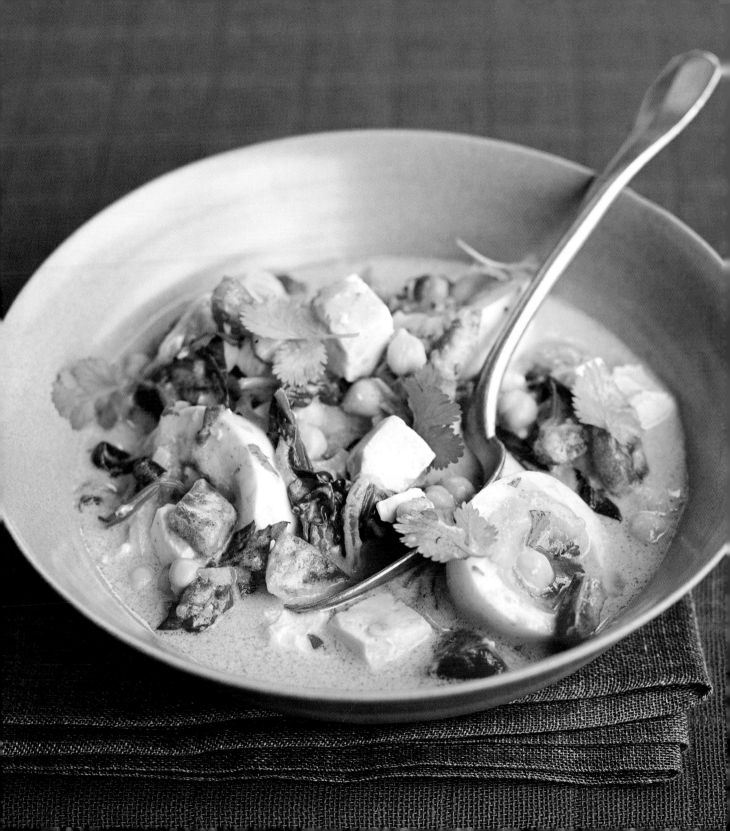

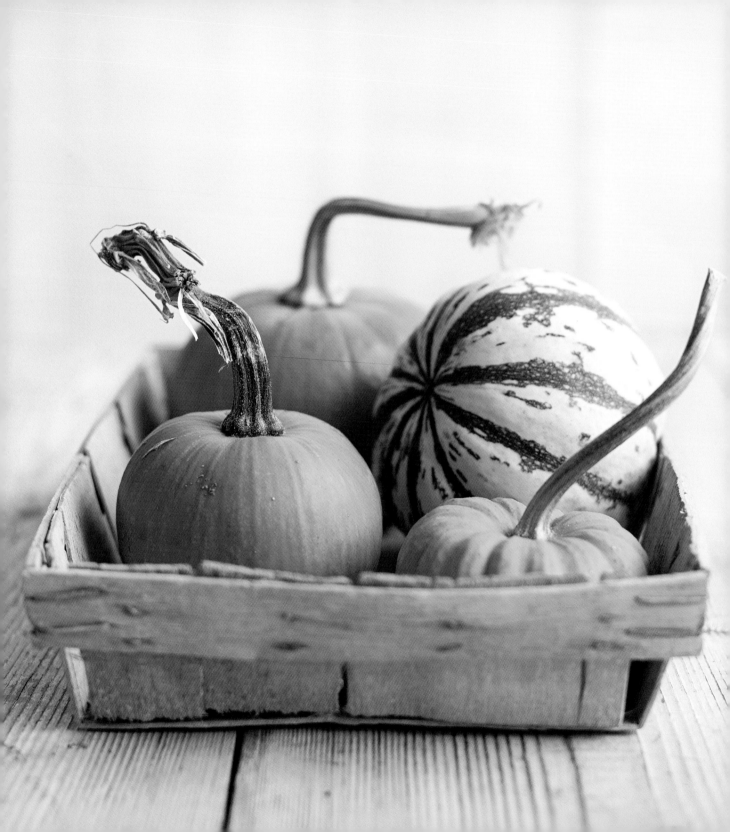

chapter four

main
courses

gnocchi with pumpkin, mushrooms and parsley

The Italians waste nothing, and from nothing create wonderful dishes of sheer brilliance. Here, stale wholemeal breadcrumbs are transformed into light, fluffy dumplings – a great vegetarian dish.

500g wholemeal flour
100g wholemeal breadcrumbs
1 tablespoon freshly grated Parmesan
2 tablespoons olive oil
½ small pumpkin, skinned, deseeded and cut into dice

300g chestnut mushrooms, thinly sliced
2 garlic cloves, crushed
2 tablespoons roughly chopped fresh parsley
freshly ground black pepper
ground nutmeg

Serves 4

In a bowl, blend the flour with the breadcrumbs and add enough warm water to form a thick but soft elastic dough. Add the Parmesan and turn out the dough onto a floured work surface. Knead the dough for 4–5 minutes until soft.

Roll out the dough into 2.5cm thick ropes, then cut these into 2cm pieces. Roll each piece into a ball and then press them with your thumb and shape them into small gnocchi.

Bring a large pan of water to the boil, add the gnocchi and simmer for 15–20 minutes – they will float to the surface of the pan. Remove with a slotted spoon and drain.

Meanwhile, heat the olive oil in a non-stick pan, add the pumpkin and cook for 4–5 minutes over a medium heat until it begins to soften. Add the mushrooms and garlic and toss with the pumpkin for about 5 minutes until cooked and golden. Add the parsley and the drained gnocchi to the pan and toss well together. Season well with black pepper and nutmeg and serve in deep pasta-style bowls.

4 PORTIONS: 524 KCALS, 21G PROTEIN, 10G FAT, 1.8G SATURATED FAT, 93G CARBOHYDRATE, 4.9G SUGAR, 14.3G FIBRE, 0.21G SALT, 84MG SODIUM

grilled tandoori vegetables

In the summer these vegetables are excellent cooked on a charcoal barbecue. Serve with a classic mint-flavoured yogurt sauce on the side.

1 teaspoon ground cumin
1 teaspoon garam masala
1 teaspoon ground coriander
¼ teaspoon ground turmeric
½ teaspoon red chilli powder
2 garlic cloves, crushed
juice of 1 lemon
little red food colouring (optional)
150ml low-fat natural yogurt
4 small onions, peeled, halved
1 celeriac, peeled and cut into large pieces.

1 small butternut squash, peeled and cut into wedges
400g baby carrots, peeled
8 baby aubergines, halved
1 large red pepper, deseeded and cut into thick strips
2 tablespoons olive oil
lemon wedges, to serve
100ml low-fat yogurt
2 tablespoons chopped fresh mint, to serve

Serves 4

Place the spices, garlic, lemon juice and food colouring, if using, into a bowl and mix to a paste with the yogurt.

Blanch the onions and celeriac in a pan of boiling water for 5 minutes, then refresh under cold water, drain well and dry. Stir into the yogurt marinade along with the remaining vegetables, rubbing the marinade well into the vegetables. Cover with clingfilm and refrigerate for 24 hours (48 hours is even better) to allow the flavours to infuse.

Heat a chargrill or grill pan. When hot, remove the vegetables from the marinade, brush over with the oil, place on the grill and cook, turning regularly to ensure even cooking and charring – it will take 20–25 minutes until the vegetables are soft and cooked through.

Serve with the lemon wedges and minted yogurt raita on the side.

4 PORTIONS: 254 KCALS, 10G PROTEIN, 9G FAT, 1.2G SATURATED FAT, 35G CARBOHYDRATE, 25.1G SUGAR, 13.2G FIBRE, 0.62G SALT, 242MG SODIUM

split pea and apricot vadas

The great thing about these little vadas is that they can be prepared in advance and frozen. Vadas are a type of savoury snack from southern India. They can vary in both shape and size, though generally they are prepared in a disc shape. Made from various pulses mixed with gram flour (chickpea), they are commonly prepared in Indian homes or sold as a snack food throughout the Indian sub-continent. Gram flour is available from health food stores. Serve with tamarind chutney.

225g yellow split peas, soaked overnight in lots of water
75g dried apricots, soaked in warm water, drained and dried
2 tablespoons gram flour
1 teaspoon cumin seeds, lightly toasted
½ teaspoon curry powder
½ teaspoon fennel seeds, lightly toasted
1 small green, chilli, deseeded and finely chopped
1 small onion, finely chopped
sunflower oil, for frying
100ml low-fat natural yogurt, to serve
tamarind chutney, to serve

Serves 4

Place the split peas and apricots in a blender, blitz in quick pulses until the mix is coarsely ground. Transfer to a bowl, add the gram flour, spices, chilli and onion and mix well together. Place in a fridge to chill for 30 minutes.

Using wet hands, divide the mixture into 24 equal-size balls, then flatten them slightly.

Heat a non-stick frying pan with 2.5cm of sunflower oil, when hot, add the vadas a few at a time and cook until golden and crispy. Drain on kitchen paper.

Place the vadas on a serving plate, drizzle with yogurt, then drizzle with the tamarind chutney. Serve.

4 PORTIONS: 293 KCALS, 15G PROTEIN, 7G FAT, 1.3G SATURATED FAT, 45G CARBOHYDRATE, 10.2G SUGAR, 5.8G FIBRE, 0.1G SALT, 39MG SODIUM

summer provençale bake

A simple Provençal-inspired bake or gratin, great as a vegetarian main course or as a vegetable to accompany a meat or fish dish. If you like you can add some reduced-fat mozzarella to the vegetables before sprinkling over the crust.

1 red onion, peeled and cut into wedges
4 medium courgettes, thickly sliced
2 aubergines, cut into 2cm cubes
2 heads fennel, trimmed, fronds removed and cut into wedges
240g Sunblush tomatoes in oil
2 garlic cloves, crushed
100g wholemeal breadcrumbs
1 tablespoon prepared pesto
1 tablespoon chopped fresh flat-leaf parsley
freshly ground black pepper

Serves 4

Preheat the oven to 200°C/400°F/gas mark 6.

Place onion, courgettes, aubergines, fennel, Sunblush tomatoes and their oil in a bowl, add the garlic and season with black pepper.

Arrange in a gratin dish large enough to take all the vegetables in a single layer. Place in the oven and bake for 30 minutes, basting regularly with juices until the vegetables are golden.

In a separate bowl, mix the crumbs, pesto and parsley. Spoon the crumb mix over the vegetables and return the dish to the oven for 5 minutes until the crust is golden.

4 PORTIONS: 435 KCALS, 10G PROTEIN, 34G FAT, 4.9G SATURATED FAT, 24G CARBOHYDRATE, 10.8G SUGAR, 7.9G FIBRE, 1.75G SALT, 690MG SODIUM

caraway roasted vegetables with chestnut polenta

This is a dish I love to serve at Christmas, served with cranberry sauce on the side. The vegetables can be changed to your preference. Some brands of polenta contain salt so always check the label.

2 red onions, quartered
4 carrots, halved lengthways
4 parsnips, thinly sliced diagonally
275g Brussels sprouts, halved
3 tablespoons olive oil
freshly ground black pepper
1 teaspoon caraway seeds

For the polenta
100g ready-cooked vacuum-packed chestnuts
1 garlic clove, crushed
2 sprigs thyme
600ml semi-skimmed milk
125g quick-cook polenta
little grated nutmeg

Serves 4

Preheat the oven to 200°C/400°F/gas mark 6.

Place the vegetables in a roasting tin, drizzle with 2 tablespoons olive oil, season with black pepper and caraway and toss together. Roast the vegetables for 45 minutes or until tender and caramelised. Meanwhile, place the chestnuts in a blender with a little water and blitz to a wet paste.

Bring the milk, garlic and thyme to the boil and simmer for 5 minutes, then remove the thyme sprigs.

Rain in the polenta a little at a time, whisking constantly at first and then using a wooden spoon as it thickens. Add the chestnut purée and season with nutmeg and black pepper. The polenta should be the consistency of wet mashed potato, slightly pourable.

Divide the polenta between 4 serving plates, top with the vegetables, drizzle with the remaining olive oil and serve.

4 PORTIONS: 459 KCALS, 14G PROTEIN, 15G FAT, 3G SATURATED FAT, 71G CARBOHYDRATE, 29.5G SUGAR, 13.5G FIBRE, 0.27G SALT, 108MG SODIUM

sweet and sour squid with cucumber and yogurt rice

Give me squid, squid and more squid, I love it! This dish is a firm favourite in our home. Crab would be lovely the same way.

650g cleaned squid, including tentacles
½ teaspoon mild curry powder
½ teaspoon ground coriander
1 tablespoon sunflower oil
1 garlic clove, crushed
4 spring onions, coarsely chopped
2 tablespoons rice wine vinegar
1 tablespoon mango chutney (finely chopped)
2 tablespoons sweet chilli sauce

40g raisins, soaked for 30 minutes, drained and dried
1 tablespoon chopped fresh mint
1 tablespoon chopped fresh coriander
¼ cucumber, peeled, halved and thickly sliced
juice of 2 limes
300g basmati rice, cooked
3 tablespoons low-fat natural yogurt
lime wedges, to garnish

Serves 4

Cut the squid into 1cm thick pieces lengthways. Place in a bowl and rub with the curry powder and ground coriander. Set aside.

Heat the oil in a non-stick wok or frying pan, add the squid, garlic and spring onions and quickly stir-fry for 1 minute. Remove to a plate.

Add the vinegar, chutney, sweet chilli sauce, raisins and herbs to the pan and cook over a high heat for 1 minute. Return the squid to the sauce, add the cucumber and lime juice and combine together.

Add the yogurt to the hot basmati rice and season with the black pepper.

Arrange the yogurt rice on serving plates, top with the squid and garnish with the lime wedges.

4 PORTIONS: 474 KCALS, 32G PROTEIN, 6G FAT, 0.5G SATURATED FAT, 77G CARBOHYDRATE, 14.4G SUGAR, 1.8G FIBRE, 0.95G SALT, 376MG SODIUM

grilled salmon with mixed peas and watercress

This dish is perfect for a summers day lunch. Lots of varying textures and extremely delicate in flavour. It is nice to garnish the dish with pea tendrils if available and some nice steamed Jersey new potatoes. If you prefer the peas can be steamed instead of boiled.

4 x 175g sustainably sourced
   skinless and boneless
   salmon fillets
3 tablespoons olive oil
freshly ground black pepper
300g snow peas, ends cut
   off and strings removed
300g sugar snap peas
250g fresh peas (podded
   weight) or use frozen

1 garlic clove, crushed
juice of ½ lemon
100g sunblush tomatoes in oil,
   drained and coarsely chopped
1 teaspoon cracked coriander
   seeds
2 tablespoons roughly chopped
   fresh coriander
bunch of watercress
fresh pea tendrils, to garnish
   (if available)

Serves 4

Preheat a chargrill or grill pan. Brush the salmon lightly with 1 tablespoon of the olive oil and season with black pepper. Place on the grill and cook for 2–3 minutes on each side.

Meanwhile, blanch the snow peas, sugar snap peas and fresh peas in a pan containing a little boiling water for 1 minute. Drain well and season with black pepper.

Heat the remaining oil in a pan with the garlic, lemon juice, tomatoes, coriander seeds and fresh coriander. Heat gently for 5 minutes to infuse the flavour.

To serve, divide the peas between 4 plates, top each with a grilled salmon fillet, spoon over a little of the tomato dressing and garnish with watercress and pea tendrils, if available. Serve immediately.

4 PORTIONS: 509 KCALS, 46G PROTEIN, 29G FAT, 5.4G SATURATED FAT, 16G CARBOHYDRATE, 8.5G SUGAR, 6.7G FIBRE, 0.26G SALT, 102MG SODIUM

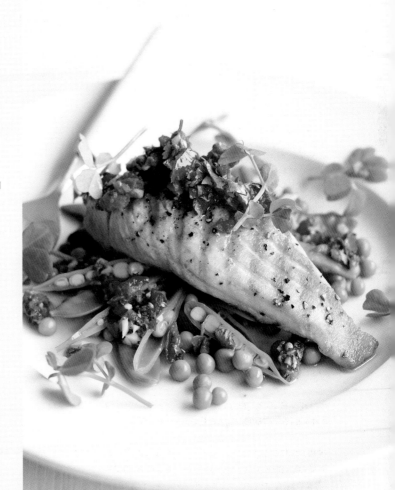

catalan tuna steaks

Tuna fish is very popular in Spain, but especially revered in Catalonia. Here the fish is topped with 'samfaina', a sort of Spanish ratatouille that makes a perfect foil for the richness of the oily tuna. The samfaina is finished with a spicy dressing, which adds a lovely bite to the sauce. I like to serve this with hot steamed new potatoes on the side.

4 x 180g sustainably sourced fresh tuna steaks
freshly ground black pepper
2 tablespoons olive oil
1 onion, cut into large dice
2 garlic cloves, crushed
2 green peppers, halved, deseeded and cut lengthways into strips
1 red pepper, halved, deseeded and cut lengthways into strips
good pinch of saffron

4 firm ripe tomatoes, cut into large dice
1 courgette, cut into large dice
1 teaspoon caster sugar

For the spiced dressing
1 tablespoon sherry vinegar
1 teaspoon paprika
¼ teaspoon red chilli flakes (or harissa)
1 tablespoon olive oil

Serves 4

Season the tuna steaks with black pepper. In a large non-stick frying pan, heat half the olive oil, add the tuna and cook for 1 minute on each side. Transfer to a plate and keep warm.

Add the remaining oil to the pan, add the onion, garlic and peppers and cook for 5 minutes until beginning to soften. Add the saffron, diced tomatoes, courgettes, sugar and 150ml water.

Return to the boil, add the tuna steaks, cover and simmer gently over the lowest heat for 2–3 minutes.

Mix the ingredients for the dressing together and stir into the cooking sauce. Transfer to a serving dish and serve immediately.

4 PORTIONS: 381 KCALS, 45G PROTEIN, 17G FAT, 3.1G SATURATED FAT, 11G CARBOHYDRATE, 9.5G SUGAR, 3.2G FIBRE, 0.25G SALT, 99MG SODIUM

baked hake with peas, lettuce and clams

A dish I love to prepare – simple and tasty. Mussels can be used instead of clams, following the same method. This is also good served with mashed potato, whipped until light and fluffy with a little good olive oil.

4 eggs
2 tablespoons olive oil
1 onion, finely chopped
2 garlic cloves, crushed
4 x 200g sustainably sourced hake steaks
600g small vongole-style fresh clams
125g fresh peas (podded weight, or use frozen)

1 little gem lettuce, shredded
3 tablespoons roughly chopped fresh flat-leaf parsley
150ml dry white wine
100ml fish stock (see page 156; if using ready-made products or stock cubes use 'low-salt' varieties)

Serves 4

Preheat the oven to 190°C/375°F/gas mark 5.

Bring a small pan of water to the boil, carefully immerse the eggs into the pan and simmer gently for 5 minutes until soft boiled. Remove, peel and keep warm.

Meanwhile heat the olive oil in an ovenproof casserole on the hob, add the onion and garlic and cook for 1–2 minutes. Place the pieces of hake on top and cook for 1–2 minutes on each side until golden.

Add the clams, peas, lettuce, parsley, white wine and stock and bring to the boil. Cover and place in the oven to braise for 6–8 minutes or until tender.

Arrange the hake on individual serving plates, then pour over the clams and braising liquor. Cut each egg in half and use to decorate the dish. Serve immediately.

4 PORTIONS: 401 KCALS, 50G PROTEIN, 18G FAT, 3.7G SATURATED FAT, 8G CARBOHYDRATE, 4.1G SUGAR, 2.2G FIBRE, 0.78G SALT, 307MG SODIUM

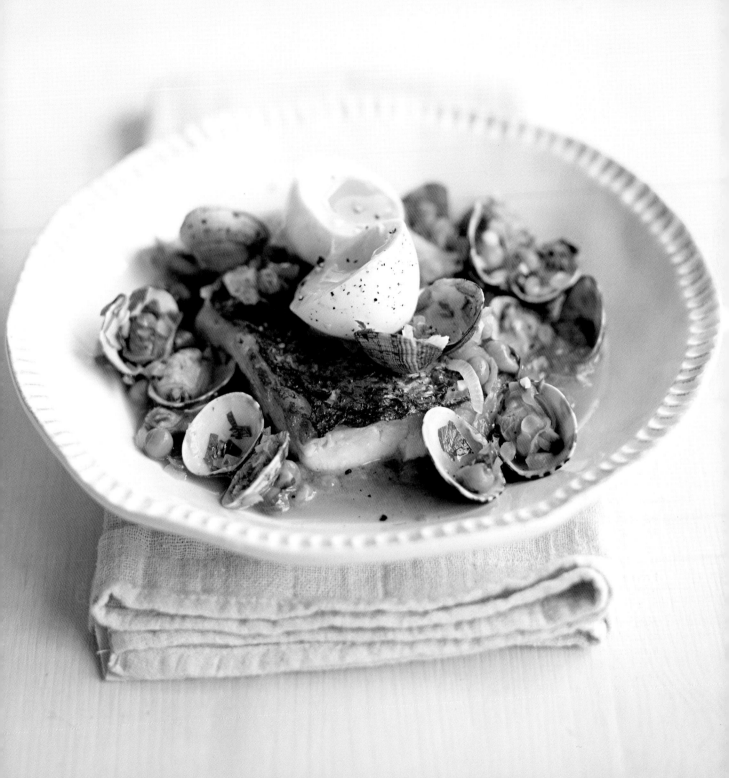

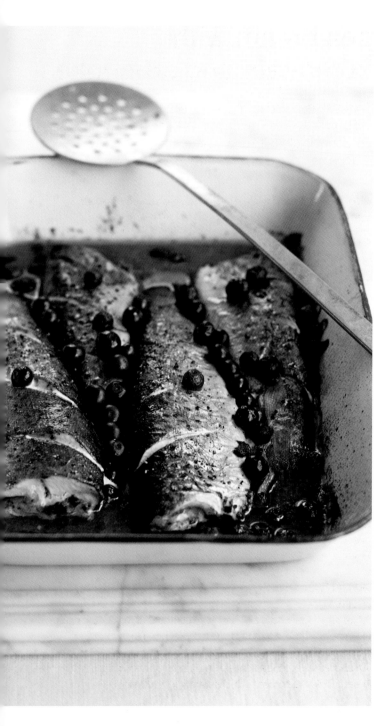

baked trout with sorrel and blueberries

The tart flavour of the sorrel works beautifully in this dish with the sweet-tasting blueberries. I serve the trout with steamed young baby carrots.

4 x 225g sustainable sourced fresh brown trout, gutted and cleaned
30g sorrel, leaves only
25g fresh flat-leaf parsley, leaves only
175g blueberries

1 garlic clove, crushed
1 tablespoon balsamic vinegar
½ teaspoon Dijon mustard

Serves 4

Preheat the oven to 190°C/375°F/gas mark 5.

With a sharp knife remove head from the fish. Slash the fish three times on each side. Place it skin side up on a work surface and gently press down the backbone to loosen it from the fish, then flip it over and ease away the backbone from the fish with your hands.

Carefully remove as many of the inner small bones as possible, then fold over the fish to its original shape. Place the sorrel and remaining ingredients (except the blueberries) in a blender or food processor and blitz to a smooth thick sauce. Season the trout with black pepper.

Place the trout in a large, lightly greased baking dish, open them up, divide the sorrel sauce between them and fold over again to conceal the sauce. Neatly return them to their original shape and scatter over the blueberries.

Cover the fish with foil and bake for 15 minutes, then uncover and cook for a further 10 minutes until the trout is cooked.

Carefully remove the fish using a fish slice and place on individual serving plates. Spoon over any excess juices from the pan and serve with steamed carrots, if desired.

4 PORTIONS: 324 KCALS, 44G PROTEIN, 14G FAT, 2.9G SATURATED FAT, 5G CARBOHYDRATE, 3.9G SUGAR, 1.2G FIBRE, 0.38G SALT, 149MG SODIUM

snapper in crazy water

A strange-sounding dish, first created by Neapolitan fishermen in Italy who cooked the fish in 'Aqua Pazza' or crazy water. I have tasted numerous variations: here is mine. For a tasty alternative, add some small clams or mussels to the broth along with the fish. Try serving the snapper on a bed of lightly sautéed spinach and cooked chickpeas in olive oil.

2 tablespoons olive oil
¼ teaspoon red chilli flakes
2 small bay leaves
2 garlic cloves, peeled and thinly sliced
50ml dry white wine
1 lemon, thinly sliced
1 anchovy fillet, soaked in water for 10 minutes, then chopped
2 tablespoons superfine baby capers, rinsed, drained
300g ripe firm tomatoes, chopped
4 x 175g sustainably sourced snapper fillets, cleaned
3 tablespoons roughly chopped fresh flat-leaf parsley

Serves 4

Place the olive oil, chilli flakes, bay leaves and garlic in a shallow casserole-style pan, cover with the wine and 400ml water and bring to the boil. Add the lemon slices, anchovies, capers and tomatoes, then reduce the heat to a simmer.

Season the fish with black pepper, then add to the broth along with the parsley – the liquid should come only halfway up the fish. Cover with a lid, reduce the heat and poach the snapper for 3–4 minutes until just tender.

Transfer the fish to deep serving bowls, pour over some of the broth and garnish to serve.

4 PORTIONS: 239 KCALS, 35.7G PROTEIN, 8.3G FAT, 1.3G SATURATED FAT, 4.6G CARBOHYDRATE, 4.1G SUGAR, 1.2G FIBRE, 0.86G SALT, 339MG SODIUM

sea bream with kumquats and artichokes

This dish is an adaptation of a similar dish I had in Paris at one of France's best-known haunts, Le Bouquinistes. If kumquats are not available, orange segments or slices would work equally well.

450g large new potatoes, cleaned and cut in half lengthwise
3 tablespoons olive oil
4 x 175g cleaned sustainably sourced sea bream fillets
1 shallot, peeled, finely chopped
60ml dry white wine
200ml reduced chicken stock (see page 156; if using ready-made products or stock cubes use 'low-salt' varieties)
1 tablespoon balsamic vinegar
freshly ground black pepper
300g cooked artichokes
2 tablespoons chopped fresh coriander
2 tablespoons pine nuts, toasted
125g kumquats, sliced

Serves 4

Preheat the oven to 190°C/375°F/gas mark 5.

Heat half the olive oil in a baking tray, add the potatoes, toss well and season with black pepper. Cook in the oven for 30–40 minutes until golden, turning often. Add the artichokes during the last 10 minutes of the cooking time. Remove from the oven, add the coriander and pine nuts and keep warm.

Heat a non-stick frying pan and add the remaining oil, when hot. Season the fish with black pepper and cook on each side until crispy, then turn and cook on the other side for a further 2 minutes. Remove from the pan and keep warm.

Add the shallot and kumquats to the pan and fry over a low heat until they are just beginning to take colour. Pour over the white wine, reduced stock and vinegar and boil for 3–4 minutes until the sauce is reduced in volume by one third.

Arrange the vegetables on serving plates, top each with a sea bream fillet, drizzle over a little sauce, then serve.

4 PORTIONS: 414 KCALS, 35G PROTEIN, 17G FAT, 2.5G SATURATED FAT, 30G CARBOHYDRATE, 6.1G SUGAR, 4.6G FIBRE, 0.56G SALT, 220MG SODIUM

chargrilled tuna with onion squash, caramelised onion and mint vinaigrette

A great dish for a summer barbecue, the vinaigrette can be made well in advance and the rest put together very quickly. I often serve this with some steamed couscous or new potatoes. Asparagus, in common with other vegetables, is a good source of potassium, which can help lower blood pressure. Onion squash is a bright orange squash similar in shape to an onion. If unavailable, use the more readily available butternut squash instead.

1 onion squash
16 asparagus tips, trimmed
1 tablespoon olive oil
1 garlic clove, crushed
1 red chilli, deseeded and finely chopped
4 x 175g sustainably sourced tuna steaks
freshly ground black pepper

For the vinaigrette
3 tablespoons olive oil
2 small red onion, finely chopped
1 tablespoon honey
2 tablespoons balsamic vinegar
2 tablespoons chopped fresh mint

Serves 4

Cut the onion squash into 12 wedges, discard the inner seeds and, using a small knife, remove the outer skin.

Cook the asparagus in a pan of boiling water for 2–3 minutes, then remove with a slotted spoon and set aside.

For the vinaigrette, heat 1 tablespoon of the olive oil in a pan, add the onion and fry for 4–5 minutes until lightly coloured and softened. Add the honey and caramelise lightly in the pan for a further 15 minutes. Remove to a bowl and cool. Add the balsamic vinegar, remaining oil and chopped mint, season with black pepper and set aside.

Preheat a chargrill or grill pan until hot. Toss the onion squash wedges and asparagus with a little oil, garlic and chilli and place the squash on the grill to cook for 10–12 minutes, then add the asparagus, cook for a further 5 minutes, or until the vegetables are golden and lightly caramelised. Remove and keep warm.

Season the tuna steaks then brush with a little olive oil. Place on the grill for 2–3 minutes until the tuna is cooked rare (a little longer if you prefer it more well done).

Place the tuna steaks on a bed of the chargrilled squash and asparagus, spoon over the onion and mint vinaigrette and serve.

4 PORTIONS: 407 KCALS, 44G PROTEIN, 19G FAT, 3.4G SATURATED FAT, 15G CARBOHYDRATE, 10.1G SUGAR, 2.5G FIBRE, 0.22G SALT, 89MG SODIUM

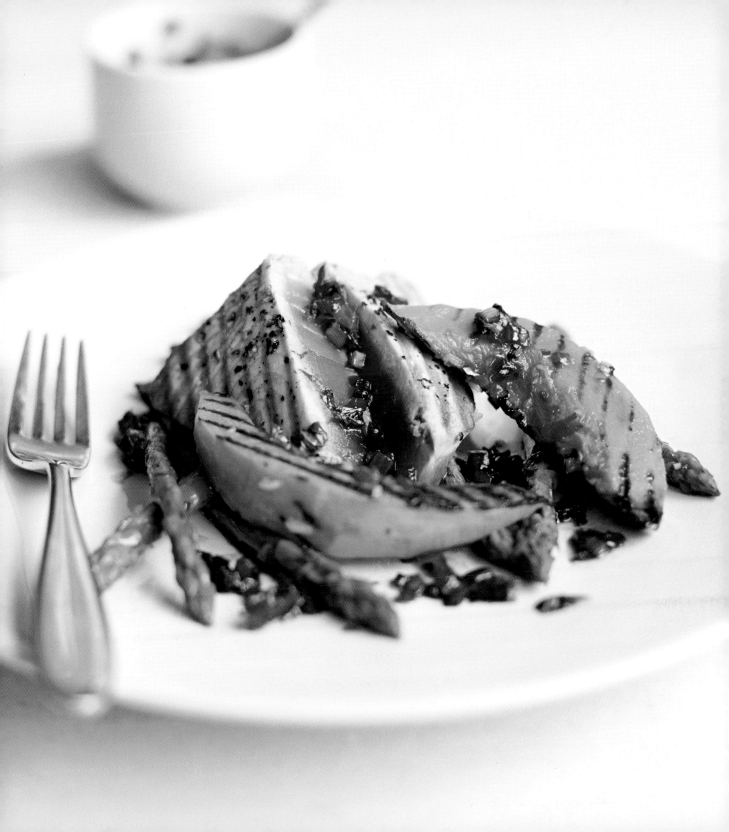

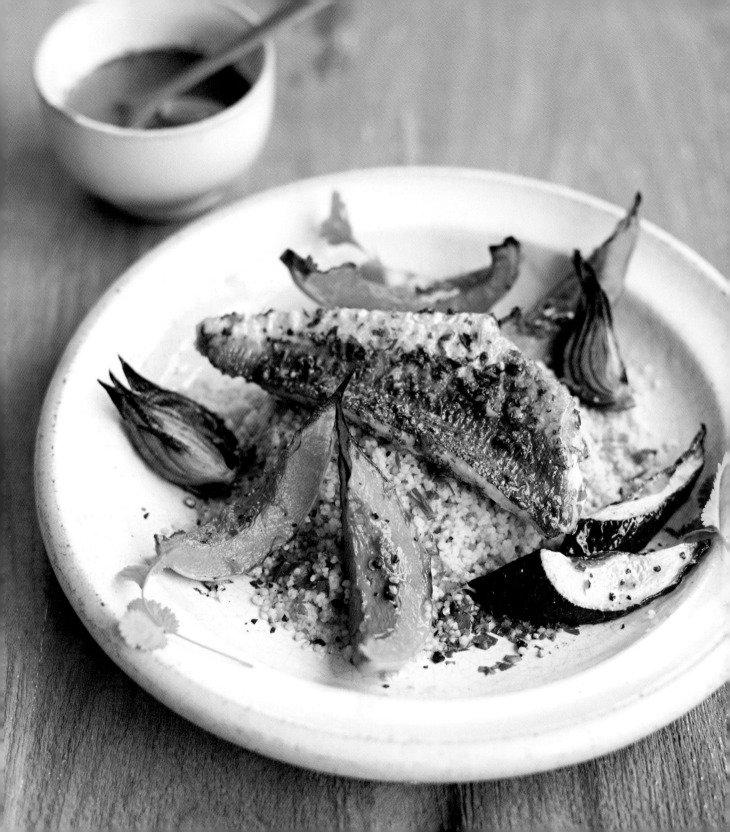

fish couscous

Couscous is the national dish of Morocco. It is a semolina grain, so is a starchy food that provides energy, fibre, vitamins and minerals. It can be served with meat or vegetables cooked in a spicy broth. This is a recipe I like to make at home, conjuring up many wonderful memories of a trip to Marrakech, such an enticing and mystical city. Serve the couscous with a selection of roasted vegetables of your choice, roasted in a touch of olive oil and seasoned with ground cumin.

4 x 175g boneless sustainably sourced
  sea trout fillets

450g quick-cook couscous
500ml boiling water or chicken stock
½ teaspoon dried chilli flakes
2 tablespoons sunflower oil
selection of vegetables for roasting,
  e.g. 200g carrots, 200g squash, 2 courgettes,
  cut in large equal-size pieces

For the marinade
1 garlic clove, crushed
2 tablespoons chopped fresh coriander
  (plus a few extra leaves to garnish)
2 tablespoons chopped fresh flat-leaf parsley
3 tablespoons olive oil
½ teaspoon ground cumin
½ teaspoon sweet paprika
¼ teaspoon cayenne pepper
¼ teaspoon ground turmeric
150ml chicken stock (see page 156; if using
  ready-made products or stock cubes use
  'low-salt' varieties)
juice of 1 small lemon

Serves 4

In a dish combine all the marinade ingredients except the chicken stock, add the trout fillets and mix well. Cover with clingfilm and marinate in the fridge overnight.

Preheat the oven to 200°C/400°F/gas mark 6 and roast the carrots and squash pieces in a little olive oil for 25 minutes. Add the courgettes and cook for a further 10 minutes until all are cooked and golden.

Place the couscous in a bowl, add the boiling water, chilli flakes and oil and stir well together. Cover with clingfilm and set aside for 5 minutes to steam. Remove the clingfilm, fluff up the couscous with a fork, cover with clingfilm again and leave to steam for a further 2 minutes. Keep warm.

Remove the fish from the marinade, place on a baking tray and bake for 6–8 minutes or until cooked.

Meanwhile, heat the stock, whisk in the marinade ingredients and bring to the boil.

Pile the couscous high on serving plates. Top with the roasted vegetables, then the sea trout fillets. Drizzle over some of the marinade broth, garnish with the extra coriander and serve.

4 PORTIONS: 600 KCALS, 42G PROTEIN, 22G FAT, 3.7G SATURATED FAT, 62G CARBOHYDRATE, 4G SUGAR, 1G FIBRE, 0.31G SALT, 122MG SODIUM

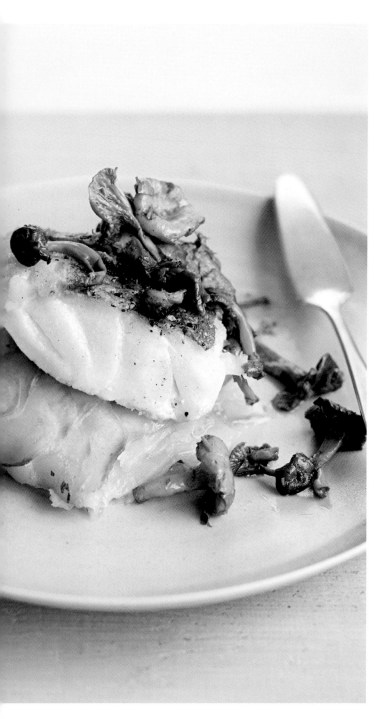

baked cod boulangère

The beauty of this dish is that the cod fillets release their juices into the potatoes when they are baked – quite delicious. Boulangère potatoes are so named because in France they were given to local bakers to place in their bread ovens after the day's baking to cook slowly.

1kg potatoes (e.g. Desirée or Maris Piper), peeled and thinly sliced
3 tablespoons olive oil, for greasing and drizzling
2 onions, thinly sliced
freshly ground black pepper
1 teaspoon chopped fresh rosemary

Serves 4

375g hot chicken stock (see page 156; if using ready-made products or stock cubes use 'low-salt' varieties)
4 x 175g sustainably sourced cod fillets, skin on
2 tablespoons olive oil
225g chanterelle mushrooms
2 tablespoons roughly chopped fresh flat-leaf parsley

Preheat the oven to 180°C/350°F/gas mark 4.

Lightly grease a large ovenproof dish with a little olive oil. Arrange layers of the potatoes and onions in the dish, seasoning each layer with black pepper and a little rosemary.

Finish with a layer of the potatoes in a neat overlapping pattern. Press down on the potatoes firmly. Pour over the hot stock to just cover the potatoes, cover with tin foil and cook in the oven for 40 minutes. Remove the foil, return to the oven to colour the potatoes for a further 20 minutes.

Season the cod with black pepper. Place the cod fillets onto the potatoes, drizzle each with a little olive oil and return the dish to the oven for 10–12 minutes to cook the fish.

To finish, heat the remaining oil in a non-stick frying pan, when hot add the mushrooms and fry for 2–3 minutes until golden. Season, add the flat-leaf parsley and mix well.

Arrange the cod and boulangère potatoes on serving plates. Spoon over the mushrooms and serve.

4 PORTIONS: 480 KCALS, 39G PROTEIN, 16G FAT, 2.3G SATURATED FAT, 48G CARBOHYDRATE, 4.5G SUGAR, 4.7G FIBRE, 0.34G SALT, 135MG SODIUM

grilled sea bream with cauliflower and caper sauce

The caper sauce adds a wonderful piquant flavour to the sea bream, and is also great served over scallops and grilled vegetables. Make it a day ahead it will help the flavours meld together beautifully.

2 tablespoons olive oil
4 x 175g sustainably sourced sea bream fillets, boneless
1 garlic clove, crushed
½ red chilli, deseeded and finely chopped
425g cauliflower florets
good pinch of saffron
2 tablespoons pine nuts, toasted
50g raisins, soaked in warm water for 30 minutes, drained and dried
freshly ground black pepper

For the sauce
2 tablespoons capers, rinsed
1 tablespoon chopped tarragon
1 tablespoon chopped flat-leaf parsley
1 small roasted red pepper, cut into small dice
1 shallot, finely chopped
1 hard-boiled egg, peeled and chopped into small pieces
3 tablespoons olive oil
juice of ½ lemon

Serves 4

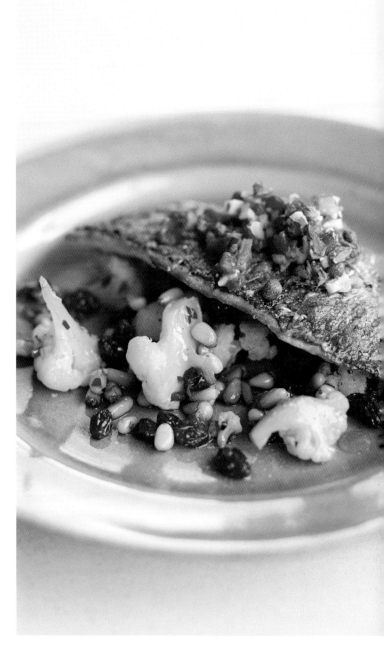

Heat 1 tablespoon of the olive oil in a non-stick pan, add the garlic, chilli and cauliflower and cook for 2 minutes. Add a little water and the saffron and cook gently until the cauliflower is cooked but still retaining its shape. Add the pine nuts and raisins and season with black pepper.

Heat a grill pan or chargrill until hot. Season the bream fillets with black pepper, brush with oil then cook, skin-side down, for 3–4 minutes, then carefully turn it over using a fish slice and cook for a further 2–3 minutes or until cooked.

Meanwhile, mix together all the ingredients for the sauce in a bowl and season with black pepper.

Arrange the cauliflower on 4 serving plates, top each with a grilled bream fillet, spoon over the caper sauce and serve.

4 PORTIONS: 424 KCALS, 38G PROTEIN, 25G FAT, 3.7G SATURATED FAT, 14G CARBOHYDRATE, 12.3G SUGAR, 3G FIBRE, 1.18G SALT, 465MG SODIUM

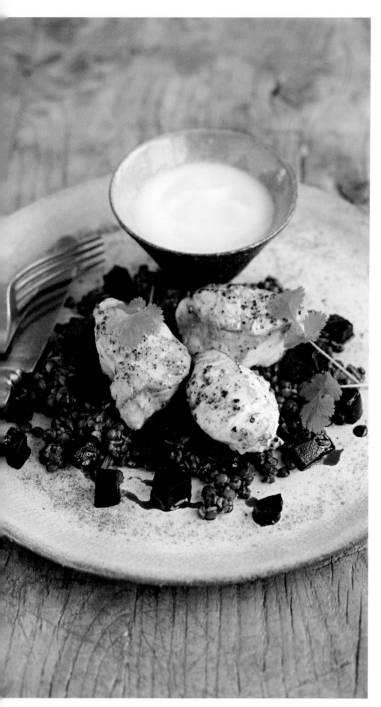

monkfish with beetroot, cumin and braised lentils

I love to serve this on a creamy olive oil mashed potato or parsnip mash, both are delicious.

2 x 150g raw beetroots, peeled and
    cut into 3cm cubes
2 tablespoons olive oil
2 shallots, finely chopped
½ teaspoon ground cumin
1 garlic clove, crushed
180g Puy lentils (or castelluces)
400ml reduced chicken stock
(see page 156; if using ready-made
    products or stock cubes use
    'low-salt' varieties)
few sprigs of thyme

4 x 150g cleaned sustainably
    sourced monkfish fillets, each
    cut into 3 equal-sized pieces
2 tablespoons sunflower oil
2 tablespoons balsamic vinegar
1 teaspoon caster sugar
2 tablespoons chopped
    fresh coriander

For the shallot purée
6 large shallots, thinly sliced
50g short-grain rice
300ml semi-skimmed milk

Serves 4

Place the beetroots in a pan, cover with water and cook for 50 minutes–1 hour until tender. Heat the olive oil in a heavy-based pan, add the shallots, cumin and garlic and sweat together for 1 minute. Add the lentils, chicken stock and thyme, bring to the boil and simmer for 30 minutes. Heat the vinegar and sugar in a pan, add the beetroot and lightly cook for 2–3 minutes until they turn to a sweet and sour flavour.

When the lentils are cooked, stir in the sweet and sour beetroot, season with black pepper and keep warm.

For the purée, blanch the shallots in a pan of boiling water for 5 minutes, then drain. Return to the pan, add the milk and rice, bring to the boil and simmer for 30 minutes. Transfer to a blender and blitz until smooth.

Season the monkfish with black pepper. Heat the oil in a non-stick frying pan, add the monkfish and cook for 3–4 minutes on each side until golden and cooked through. Arrange the fish on 4 individual serving plates, garnish with the beetroot, lentils and shallot purée and serve immediately.

4 PORTIONS: 458 KCALS, 41G PROTEIN, 14G FAT, 2.4G SATURATED FAT, 44G CARBOHYDRATE, 12.3G SUGAR, 5.8G FIBRE, 0.35G SALT, 139MG SODIUM

roasted skate with fruit and vegetable sauce

Skate has to be very fresh to enjoy it at its best: as a rule I like to consume it within eight hours of purchasing, as old skate can release an ammonia like smell and flavour which is very unpleasant. When fresh it can be a revelation.

1 Granny Smith apple, peeled and cored
1 small mango, peeled
150g freshly prepared pineapple
1 small red pepper, halved and deseeded
2 sticks celery, trimmed
2 tablespoons rapeseed oil
4 x 275g sustainably sourced skate wings

freshly ground black pepper
juice of 1 lemon
2 tablespoons sherry vinegar
2 teaspoons brown sugar
100ml tomato juice (no added salt)
1 tablespoon baby capers, rinsed and drained
2 tablespoons chopped fresh flat-leaf parsley

Serves 4

Cut the apple, mango and pineapple into 2cm dice. Cut the celery and red pepper into pieces the same size and set aside.

Heat 1 tablespoon of the oil in a large non-stick frying pan. Season the skate wings with black pepper and add to the pan. Cook the skate over a medium heat for 3–4 minutes each side until crisp and golden. When cooked transfer to a plate and keep warm.

Return the pan to the heat, add the prepared fruit and vegetables and sweat for 2 minutes. Add the sherry vinegar, sugar and tomato juice and simmer for 1 minute. Finally add the capers and parsley and season with black pepper.

Steam the spinach for 2 minutes and season with black pepper. Arrange on a plate, place the skate on top, spoon over the sauce and serve.

4 PORTIONS: 267 KCALS, 32G PROTEIN, 7G FAT, 0.5G SATURATED FAT, 21G CARBOHYDRATE, 20.1G SUGAR, 3.5G FIBRE, 1.02G SALT, 402MG SODIUM

cioppino (seafood stew)

Often spelt 'Ciuppin', this seafood stew is said to have originated on the west coast of America, off San Francisco. The word ciuppin means chopped in Italian and it is said the fisherman made the stew on board their vessel while at sea, using chopped fish.

2 tablespoons olive oil
1 head fennel, thinly sliced
1 onion, chopped
1 garlic clove, crushed
½ teaspoon red chilli flakes
600g mixed fish (e.g. snapper, halibut, mullet), cut into large pieces
60ml dry white wine
275ml fish stock (see page 156; if using ready-made products or stock cubes use 'low-salt' varieties)
400g can chopped tomatoes (no added salt)
12 raw prawns, peeled and deveined
50ml Pernod
2 tablespoons chopped fresh flat-leaf parsley

Serves 4

In a shallow heavy-based pan, heat the oil, add the fennel, onion and garlic and cook over a low heat for 8–10 minutes until softened and lightly caramelised.

Add the chilli flakes and fish pieces and place on top of the fennel. Pour over the wine, boil for 1 minute, add the fish stock and tomatoes and bring to a simmer. Add the prawns and Pernod and simmer for a further 5 minutes. Stir in the parsley and serve immediately.

4 PORTIONS: 343 KCALS, 37G PROTEIN, 15G FAT, 2.6G SATURATED FAT, 7G CARBOHYDRATE, 5.1G SUGAR, 2.7G FIBRE, 0.72G SALT, 284MG SODIUM

grilled sea bass with lemongrass and ginger pesto

An oriental twist on the Italian classic 'pesto' sauce. I serve the bass on grilled slices of courgettes but asparagus is also good with the dish. Marinating fish in lime or lemon juice before cooking helps avoid the need to add salt for flavour.

4 x 175g cleaned sustainably sourced sea bass fillets
juice of 1 lime
2 tablespoons olive oil
freshly ground black pepper
400g cut courgettes, sliced thickly on the bias

For the pesto
2 sticks lemongrass, outer husks removed, inner very finely chopped
5cm piece root ginger, peeled and finely chopped
1 garlic clove, crushed
15 fresh basil leaves
small bunch fresh coriander leaves
25g unsalted roasted peanuts
4 tablespoons sunflower oil

Serves 4

Place the sea bass in a shallow dish, season with black pepper, pour over the lime juice with the olive oil and leave to marinate for 1 hour at room temperature.

To cook the courgettes, heat a grill pan until very hot. Season the thick-cut slices of courgettes with black pepper and cook on the grill for 4–5 minutes, turning them regularly until cooked and golden.

For the pesto, place all the ingredients in a small blender and blitz to a coarse purée. Heat a chargrill or grill pan, add the sea bass fillets and cook for 3–4 minutes, skin-side down, until golden and crispy. Carefully turn over and cook for a further 2 minutes.

Arrange the sea bass fillets on a bed of grilled courgette slices and top with the oriental pesto sauce.

4 PORTIONS: 337 KCALS, 38G PROTEIN, 19G FAT, 3G SATURATED FAT, 4G CARBOHYDRATE, 2.3G SUGAR, 1.3G FIBRE, 0.32G SALT, 124MG SODIUM

fish korma

Traditionally, whenever I make a chicken-style korma, I always use coconut cream. However, in this Bengali-style variation that uses fish I prefer to use yogurt, which makes the sauce a little more tart in flavour but also lower in saturated fat. Most types of fish work well here; salmon, halibut or cod. Serve with steamed or boiled basmati rice – a simple but impressive dish for all to enjoy.

5cm piece root ginger, peeled
4 garlic cloves, peeled
150ml low-fat natural yogurt
1 tablespoon plain flour
1 teaspoon sugar
1kg sustainably sourced firm white fish fillets, cut into 5cm cubes
4 tablespoons sunflower oil
2 onions, chopped
½ teaspoon ground turmeric
½ teaspoon red chilli powder
1 tablespoon ground coriander
1 tablespoon ground cumin
6 whole cardamom pods, crushed
4cm piece cinnamon stick
50g ground almonds
2 tablespoons chopped coriander to garnish

Serves 4

Place the ginger and garlic in a blender, add 4 tablespoons water and blitz to a smooth paste. In a bowl, mix together the yogurt and flour, then stir in the ginger paste. Add the fish, cover with clingfilm and refrigerate for 1 hour.

Heat the oil in a heavy-based non-stick pan, add the onions and cook until lightly golden. Add the spices and cook gently for 3–4 minutes.

Remove the fish from the fridge, and add both the fish and the marinade to the pan. Increase the heat, add 300ml water and carefully bring to the boil. Add the sugar and almonds, reduce the heat and cook gently for 10–12 minutes, stirring occasionally.

Transfer to a serving plate, sprinkle over the coriander to garnish and serve with basmati rice.

4 PORTIONS: 463 KCALS, 53G PROTEIN, 22G FAT, 2.6G SATURATED FAT, 15G CARBOHYDRATE, 7G SUGAR, 1.9G FIBRE, 0.5G SALT, 196MG SODIUM

vietnamese-style snapper

Vietnam is a wonderful haven of great culture and food. It is always light, fragrant and clean tasting. This dish is no exception, embodying the virtues of quick simple and delicious, whether for a simple family meal or a dinner party main course. Lovely served with some steamed or stir-fried Asian greens.

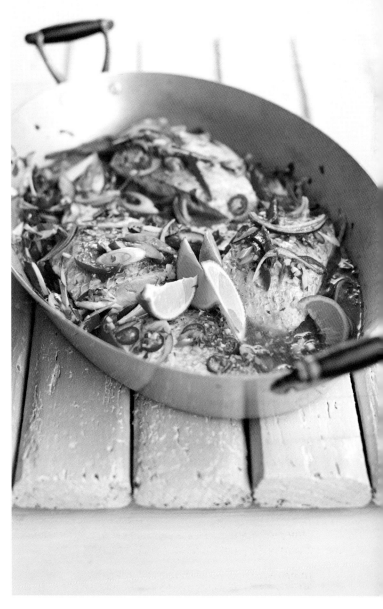

4 x 175g sustainably sourced snapper fillets, cleaned, boneless
1 tablespoon sunflower oil
1 teaspoon sesame oil
2 garlic cloves, crushed
juice of 2 limes
2 sticks lemongrass, outer leaves removed, tender inner core chopped
1 red chilli, finely sliced
1 tablespoon rice wine vinegar
2 tablespoons sweet chilli sauce
150ml chicken stock (see page 156; if using ready-made products or stock cubes use 'low-salt' varieties)
1 teaspoon reduced-salt soy sauce
2 red peppers, deseeded and cut lengthways into strips
1 red onion, thinly sliced
4 spring onions, thickly sliced on bias
3 tablespoons roughly chopped fresh coriander

Serves 4

Place the snapper fillets in a shallow dish, pour over both oils, add the garlic, lime juice, lemongrass and chilli and rub well into the fish. Cover with clingfilm and leave to marinate for 1 hour at room temperature.

Heat the vinegar and sweet chilli sauce in a large, deep-sided non-stick frying pan. When hot, add the chicken stock, soy sauce, peppers, onion, spring onions and coriander, reduce the heat and cook for 5 minutes.

Add the marinated snapper fillets and spoon over the sauce. Cover the pan with a lid and simmer for 4–5 minutes, basting the fish occasionally with the sauce.

To serve, arrange the fish on serving plates, pour over the braising sauce and garnish with a little coriander and lime.

4 PORTIONS: 250 KCALS, 36.1G PROTEIN, 6.5G FAT, 1G SATURATED FAT, 12.6G CARBOHYDRATE, 11G SUGAR, 1 8G FIBRE, 0.83G SALI, 327MG SODIUM

braised chicken in vinegar sauce

A lovely way to enjoy chicken pieces, slowly braised in a sauce made from cider vinegar, delicately flavoured with Dijon mustard.

8 chicken thighs, skin removed
freshly ground black pepper
2 tablespoons sunflower oil
4 garlic cloves, crushed
3 shallots, peeled and finely chopped
150ml cider vinegar (or white wine vinegar)
2 tablespoons honey
100ml dry white wine
200ml reduced low-salt chicken stock (see
    page 156; if using ready-made products or
    stock cubes use 'low-salt' varieties)
2 teaspoons 'no salt' tomato purée
1 teaspoon Dijon mustard
1 tablespoon chopped tarragon

Serves 4

Season the chicken thighs with black pepper. Heat the sunflower oil in a heavy-based casserole, add the chicken pieces and fry for 5–6 minutes until golden, turning regularly. Transfer to a plate.

Remove any excess fat from the pan, add the garlic and shallots and cook for 2–3 minutes until softened. Add the vinegar, honey and white wine and reduce by half in volume. Add the stock, bring to the boil, return the chicken to the pan and cook for 10–15 minutes.

Mix the tomato purée with the Dijon mustard and stir into the sauce. When the chicken is cooked, add the tarragon and season with black pepper. The sauce should be slightly tart in flavour, if necessary add a tablespoon more vinegar, then serve.

4 PORTIONS: 318 KCALS, 37G PROTEIN, 10G FAT, 2.5G SATURATED FAT, 12G CARBOHYDRATE, 11.1G SUGAR, 0.3G FIBRE, 0.54G SALT, 214MG SODIUM

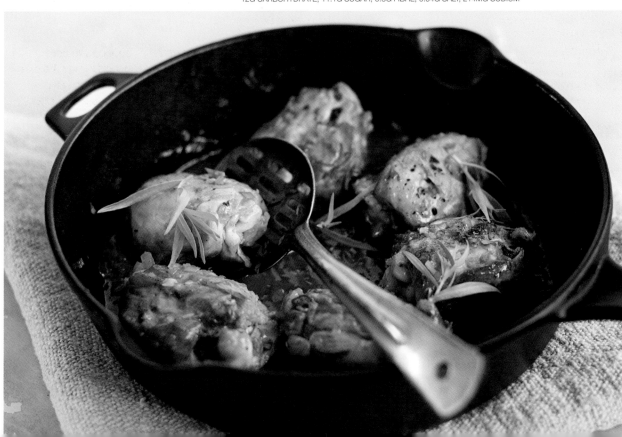

baby chicken spatchcock with lemon and herbs

This is a lovely way to cook these tender young chickens. Ask your butcher to prepare them spatchcock style. That means the backbone and breast bones removed to give a toad like appearance. The flavouring of the lemon and herbs with the delicate meat is magical. Sweet and sour root vegetables are my preferred way to serve them.

1 garlic clove, crushed
2 tablespoons chopped fresh mixed herbs
   (i.e. thyme, rosemary, flat-leaf parsley)
½ lemon, thinly sliced
4 baby chicken (450g each) prepared
   spatchcock, skin removed
2 tablespoons olive oil
200ml reduced chicken stock (see page 156;
   if using ready-made products or stock
   cubes use 'low-salt' varieties)
freshly ground black pepper
300g young carrots, peeled
300g young parsnips, peeled and halved
   lengthways
2 tablespoons chopped fresh mint
1 tablespoon olive oil
1 tablespoon maple syrup
1 tablespoon balsamic vinegar

Serves 4

Preheat the oven to 200°C/400°F/gas mark 6.

In a bowl, mix the garlic and herbs. Cut one half of the lemon into thin slices.

Lay the chicken out in a large baking tray and season with pepper. Using a small sharp knife, make small incisions over the chicken, then rub the garlic and herb mix into the slots. Lay a slice or two of lemon on each spatchcock and drizzle over the olive oil. Roast for 18–20 minutes until chicken is cooked through.

Meanwhile, blanch the carrots and parsnips in boiling water for 2 minutes, then drain. Place in another baking tin, drizzle over the olive oil and maple syrup and roast until golden and lightly caramelised, about 20 minutes. Towards the end of the cooking, add the mint and balsamic vinegar and season. Keep hot.

When the chicken is cooked, remove from baking tray and set aside. Add the reduced stock to the cooking pan, place on a high heat and stir in any residue that has caramelised on the bottom of the tin. Boil for 2 minutes and season with pepper.

Place the roasted vegetables on serving plates, top each with a roasted spatchcock chicken, pour over the pan juices and serve.

4 PORTIONS: 374 KCALS, 46G PROTEIN, 14G FAT, 2.5G SATURATED FAT, 18G CARBOHYDRATE, 11.7G SUGAR, 5.3G FIBRE, 0.5G SALT, 198MG SODIUM

hazelnut chicken with leeks and mushroom vinaigrette

If wild mushrooms are not available, portobellos make a good alternative.

1 egg
4 x 175g skinless chicken
 breasts, bone on
60g ground hazelnuts
2 tablespoons sunflower oil
400g leeks, washed and
 roughly shredded

For the vinaigrette
1 tablespoon sunflower oil
300g wild mushrooms, cleaned

1 shallot, finely chopped
1 tablespoon sherry vinegar
100ml reduced chicken stock
 (see page 156; if using ready-
 made products or stock
 cubes use 'low-salt' varieties)
1 tablespoon olive oil
2 tablespoons hazelnut oil
1 tablespoon chopped
 flat-leaf parsley

Serves 4

Beat the egg with 1 tablespoon water in a shallow dish. Dip the chicken breasts in this, then press down into the ground hazelnuts to ensure they stick to the breasts.

Heat 1 tablespoon of the oil in a non-stick frying pan, add the leeks and 100ml water, cover, reduce the heat and cook for 8–10 minutes until the leeks are tender. Drain and keep warm.

Return the pan to the heat and add another 1 tablespoon of the oil. When hot, add the chicken breast and cook for 4–5 minutes on each side until the chicken is cooked and the nutty coating is golden.

For the vinaigrette, heat another small non-stick frying pan. When hot add the sunflower oil, mushrooms and shallots and cook for 1–2 minutes until golden. Add the vinegar and stock and boil for 2 minutes. Stir in the hazelnut and olive oils, add the parsley and season with black pepper.

Arrange the leeks on serving plates, pour over the mushroom vinaigrette, top with a nut-coated cooked chicken breast and serve.

4 PORTIONS: 491 KCALS, 49G PROTEIN, 30G FAT, 3.7G SATURATED FAT, 5G CARBOHYDRATE, 3.1G SUGAR, 3.8G FIBRE, 0.4G SALT, 158MG SODIUM

braised chicken with squash, saffron and mint

A simple dish I often like to prepare at home with a Moroccan feel and delicate flavour. Always buy the best quality olives available within your price range with the least amount of salt, I find many are over salted and lack any real flavour.

750ml chicken stock (see page
 156; if using ready-made
 products or stock cubes use
 'low-salt' varieties)
good pinch of fresh saffron
 (or powdered)
12 chicken thighs, skins removed
freshly ground black pepper
1 tablespoon wholemeal flour
2 tablespoons olive oil

1 small butternut squash,
 peeled and cubed
350g baby onions, peeled
1 lemon, thinly sliced
1 garlic clove, crushed
2 teaspoons honey
12 pitted green olives
2 tablespoons chopped mint
couscous, to serve

Serves 4

Preheat the oven to 190°C/375°F/gas mark 5. Heat the stock and saffron together in a pan for 10 minutes to infuse.

Season the chicken thighs with black pepper, then dust liberally in the flour. Heat the oil in a heavy-based casserole dish on the stove, add the chicken pieces and fry until lightly golden all over. Remove and set aside.

Add the diced squash, onions, lemon slices and garlic to the casserole and lightly fry until golden. Add the saffron stock and stir well to form a light sauce around the vegetables.

Return the chicken pieces to the sauce, add the honey and olives, cover with a lid and place in the oven to cook for 15–20 minutes until the chicken is cooked through. Stir the mint into the sauce, and serve with couscous.

4 PORTIONS: 434 KCALS, 58G PROTEIN, 14G FAT, 3.6G SATURATED FAT, 20G CARBOHYDRATE, 12.1G SUGAR, 4.1G FIBRE, 1.19G SALT, 467MG SODIUM

burmese chicken

In this Burmese recipe the chicken is marinated in yogurt and spices, similar to an Indian tandoori. The yogurt makes the dish wonderfully succulent and tender.

4 x 175g skinless chicken breasts
100ml low-fat natural yogurt
1 tablespoon reduced salt soy sauce
½ teaspoon ground turmeric
1 tablespoon ground cumin
1 tablespoon ground cardamom
1 teaspoon chilli powder
2.5cm piece root ginger, peeled and chopped
1 tablespoon sunflower oil
1 garlic clove, crushed
lime wedges, to garnish

For the tomato and ginger sauce
1 tablespoon sunflower oil
4 medium ripe firm plum tomatoes, chopped
2.5cm piece root ginger, peeled and chopped
1 small green chilli, chopped
1 garlic clove, crushed
2 tablespoons roughly chopped fresh coriander
150ml tomato juice
juice of ½ lime

Serves 4

Place the chicken breasts in a dish. Combine the yogurt, soy sauce, turmeric, cumin, cardamom, chilli and ginger in a small bowl and mix thoroughly together. Whisk in the oil and garlic, then pour over the chicken breasts. Mix well to ensure the chicken is well coated with the marinade. Place in the fridge for at least 6 hours, preferably overnight

Preheat the oven to 180°C/350°F/gas mark 4.

For the sauce, heat the oil in a non-stick saucepan, add the tomatoes, ginger, chilli, garlic and coriander and sweat for 8–10 minutes until vegetables have softened. Add the tomato juice, cook for a further 10 minutes, then strain through a sieve into a clean pot. Season with black pepper, stir in the lime juice and keep warm.

Place the chicken breasts on a baking tray and bake for about 25 minutes until tender and cooked through.

Arrange the cooked chicken on serving plates, garnish with the lime wedges and serve with the sauce. Wholegrain rice makes a nice simple accompaniment.

4 PORTIONS: 308 KCALS, 45.9G PROTEIN, 9G FAT, 1.6G SATURATED FAT, 11.1G CARBOHYDRATE, 6.2G SUGAR, 1.2G FIBRE, 1.02G SALT, 394MG SODIUM

chicken with fennel, prunes and balsamic honey

For me there are few vegetables that taste equally as delicious raw as it is cooked as fennel. Raw it is crisp, assertively aromatic and fresh, while cooked, its texture and taste are transformed into something altogether different, almost more bold and delicate.

4 x 175g skinless chicken breasts
freshly ground black pepper
2 tablespoons sunflower oil
4 small-medium fennel, trimmed and cut into wedges
250g frozen (or vacuum-packed) chestnuts
1 small bay leaf
3 teaspoons balsamic vinegar
2 tablespoons honey
200ml reduced chicken stock (see page 156; if using ready-made products or stock cubes use 'low-salt' varieties)

225g ready-to-eat prunes

Serves 4

Season the chicken breasts with black pepper. Heat the oil in a non-stick frying pan, add the chicken breasts and fry until golden on both sides. Remove from the pan.

Add the fennel, chestnuts and bay leaf to the pan and cook for 5 minutes until lightly golden, turning the fennel often. Pour over the balsamic vinegar and honey to coat the fennel and chestnuts. Cook for a further 4–5 minutes to infuse the flavours.

Add the stock, prunes and chicken, cover and cook over a low heat for 10–12 minutes until the chicken is cooked through and the braising liquid forms a light sauce. Remove the bayleaf and adjust the seasoning before serving.

4 PORTIONS: 463 KCALS, 46G PROTEIN, 10G FAT, 1.7G SATURATED FAT, 51G CARBOHYDRATE, 31.9.1G SUGAR, 8.8G FIBRE, 0.36G SALT, 143MG SODIUM

chicken with pineapple, ginger and lime

The combination of chicken and pineapple is nothing new; it is prepared throughout Asia and the Caribbean to great effect. This is my variation of a dish I had in the Caribbean while working on the French island of St Martin. I prefer to use chicken legs separated into thigh and drumstick, but you could use breast of course.

4 large chicken thighs, skin removed
4 large chicken drumsticks, skin removed
freshly ground black pepper
pinch of cinnamon
pinch of turmeric
½ teaspon mild curry powder
½ teaspoon red chilli flakes
2 tablespoons sunflower oil
4 spring onions, finely chopped
juice of 2 limes

300g fresh pineapple, cut into cubes (prepared weight)
4cm piece root ginger
300ml pineapple juice (no added sugar)
300ml reduced chicken stock (see page 156; if using ready-made products or stock cubes use 'low-salt' varieties)
4 medium tomatoes, blanched, deseeded and chopped

Serves 4

Preheat the oven to 180°C/350°F/gas mark 4.

Place the chicken pieces in a dish, season with the black pepper, cinnamon, curry powder and chilli flakes, cover with clingfilm and marinate overnight in the fridge.

Heat the oil in a large flameproof casserole, add the chicken pieces and cook until brown all over. Pour off the excess oil, add the remaining ingredients, bring to the boil, cover and place in the oven for up to 40 minutes or until the chicken is tender and the sauce reduced and slightly thickened. Serve immediately with wholegrain rice.

4 PORTIONS: 330 KCALS, 39G PROTEIN, 11G FAT, 2.6G SATURATED FAT, 20G CARBOHYDRATE, 18.7G SUGAR, 2G FIBRE, 0.49G SALT, 191MG SODIUM

rabbit cacciatore

'Cacciatore' in Italian means hunter's style, and this dish, popular throughout Italy, is traditionally made with chicken. Rabbit makes a great alternative and again is one of those underestimated meats that seems to be making a little comeback, especially in the restaurant world. Also in this recipe I use porcini instead of button mushrooms, which adds another dimension to the dish. If unavailable use any type of common mushrooms. I recommend you serve this dish with creamy polenta in true Italian style.

4 large rabbit legs (or 8 large thighs)
freshly ground black pepper
pinch of dried oregano
1 tablespoon wholemeal flour
2 tablespoons olive oil
1 garlic clove, crushed
1 onion, chopped
2 red peppers, deseeded and cut into 2.5cm cubes
300g porcini (or other) mushrooms
100ml dry white wine

1 x 200g can tomatoes (no added salt)
1 tablespoon tomato purée (no added salt)
2 teaspoons caster sugar
400ml chicken stock (see page 156; if using ready-made stock or cubes use 'low salt' varieties)
10 fresh basil leaves

Serves 4

Season the rabbit with black pepper, rub all over with the dried oregano, then sprinkle over the flour.

Heat the olive oil in a large heavy-based pan, add the rabbit legs and fry until golden. Remove and set aside.

Add the garlic, onion, peppers and mushrooms to the pan and cook in the residue left in the pan. Add the white wine and boil for 2–3 minutes before adding the tomatoes, tomato purée, sugar and stock. Return to the boil.

Transfer the rabbit legs back to the sauce, cover and simmer for 40–45 minutes until the rabbit is tender. Stir the basil leaves into the sauce and cook for a further 2 minutes. Adjust seasoning and serve on a bed of creamy polenta.

4 PORTIONS: 390 KCALS, 42G PROTEIN, 16G FAT, 4.8G SATURATED FAT, 19G CARBOHYDRATE, 14.9G SUGAR, 2.8G FIBRE, 0.4G SALT, 156MG SODIUM

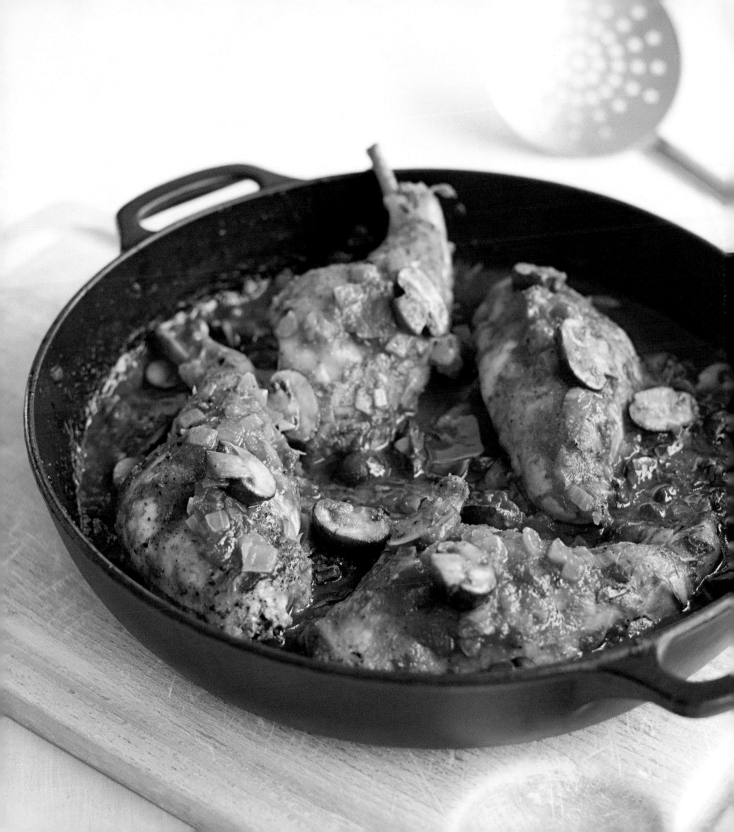

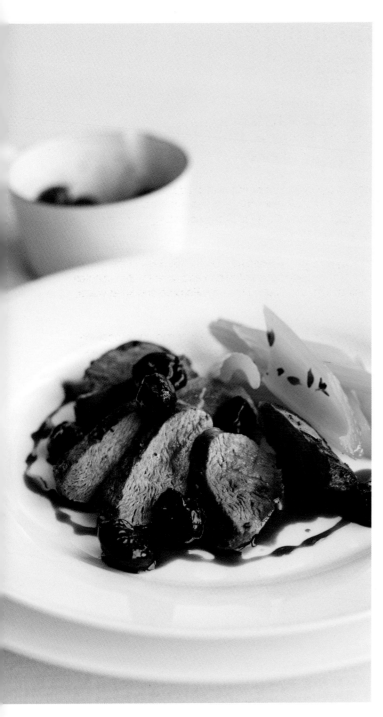

duck with cinnamon cherries and braised celery

Duck with cherries is a classic of French cuisine. By removing the duck's skin you remove a lot of the fat – the breast itself is quite lean.

1 tablespoon sunflower oil
4 x 175g boneless and skinless
    duck breasts
250g fresh or frozen cherries,
    stoned
2 teaspoons reduced-sugar
    redcurrant jelly
100ml red wine
pinch of ground cinnamon
50ml Madeira
50ml reduced chicken stock (see
    page 156; if using ready-made
    products or stock cubes use
    'low-salt' varieties)

For the celery
150ml chicken stock (see
    page 156; if using ready-made
    products or stock cubes use
    'low-salt' varieties)
few springs of thyme
1 small bunch of celery, peeled
    and cut on the bias into
    5cm lengths
freshly ground black pepper

Serves 4

To braise the celery, bring the chicken stock and thyme to the boil, cook for 5 minutes, then lower the heat, add the celery and lightly braise under a lid for 5 minutes until the celery is just cooked and the stock almost evaporated. Season and keep warm.

Heat the oil in a non-stick frying pan, add the duck breasts and cook for 4–5 minutes on each side over a medium heat until golden, a little longer if you don't want your duck pink. Remove from the pan and keep warm on a plate under foil.

Using the pan used for cooking the duck, add the cherries and redcurrant jelly and cook for 1 minute. Pour in the red wine, cinnamon, Madeira and reduced chicken stock and simmer gently for 5–6 minutes until the sauce has reduced by half. Season with black pepper.

Thickly slice the duck and place on serving plates. Pour the cherry sauce over the duck and serve with the braised celery.

4 PORTIONS: 345 KCALS, 36G PROTEIN, 14G FAT, 3.4G SATURATED FAT, 10G CARBOHYDRATE, 10.1G SUGAR, 1.7G FIBRE, 0.67G SALT, 265MG SODIUM

guinea fowl with green peppercorn sauce and gingered carrots

Guinea fowl, which tastes like slightly gamey chicken, makes a great alternative to chicken. Green peppercorns are purchased preserved in brine – simply rinse them well under cold water before use to wash away some of the salt. Some tenderstem broccoli would also go beautifully with the dish.

400g young carrots, peeled and cut in half
  lengthways if big
1 tablespoon honey
5cm piece root ginger, peeled and finely
  chopped or grated
1 tablespoon sunflower oil
4 x 175g guinea fowl breasts, skins removed
freshly ground black pepper
60ml dry white wine
2 teaspoons caster sugar
150ml pink grapefruit juice (preferably fresh)
300ml reduced chicken stock (see page 156;
  if using ready-made products or stock cubes
  use 'low-salt' varieties)
1 tablespoon green peppercorns in brine,
  rinsed and drained

Serves 4

Place the carrots in a pan, just cover with water, add the honey and ginger and bring to the boil. Reduce the heat and simmer until the carrots are just cooked and almost all the liquid has gone, leaving them in a gingery syrupy glaze. Keep warm.

Heat a non-stick frying pan and when hot add the oil. Season the guinea fowl breasts with black pepper, add to the pan and cook for 3–4 minutes on each side until golden and cooked through. Remove and keep warm, covered with foil.

Return the pan to the heat, add the wine and sugar and cook together for 2 minutes. Add the grapefruit juice and stock and boil for 5 minutes until the sauce is reduced by one-third in volume.

Strain through a fine sieve, add the green peppercorns and season to taste.

To serve arrange the cooked carrots on serving plates, top each with a cooked guinea fowl breast and pour over the sauce. Serve with steamed new potatoes, if desired.

4 PORTIONS: 354 KCALS, 40G PROTEIN, 9G FAT, 1.8G SATURATED FAT, 27G CARBOHYDRATE, 18.3G SUGAR, 2.5G FIBRE, 0.74G SALT, 293MG SODIUM

grilled duck steak with herb vinaigrette

Serving vinaigrettes as sauces for hot dishes is becoming increasingly popular. It is light and often more flavoursome than a contrived sauce, simple to put together and healthy as it's lower in fat.

1 teaspoon black peppercorns
1 teaspoon green peppercorns in brine, rinsed and drained
1 teaspoon pink peppercorns in brine, rinsed and drained
4 x 180g skinless duck breasts
100ml reduced chicken stock (see page 156; if using ready-made products or stock cubes use 'low-salt' varieties)
2 small shallots, finely chopped
1 teaspoon thyme leaves

1 tablespoon chopped fresh tarragon
1 tablespoon chopped fresh flat-leaf parsley
1 tablespoon balsamic vinegar
4 tablespoons olive oil
2 garlic cloves, crushed
225g wild mushrooms (or other mushrooms), cleaned
100g sunblush tomatoes in oil, drained and dried
100g cooked peas

Serves 4

Place the peppercorns in a mortar (or spice grinder) and pound to a coarse paste. Rub this paste liberally all over the duck breasts and leave to marinate for 30 minutes.

Heat the stock with the shallot, herbs and vinegar. Whisk in 2 tablespoons of the olive oil, bring to the boil, then remove from the heat and keep warm.

Heat a grill pan or chargrill. Brush the duck all over with 1 tablespoon of the oil and cook for 4–5 minutes on each side for medium, longer if you prefer your duck more well done. Remove the duck to a plate, cover with foil and keep warm to rest the duck.

Meanwhile, heat the remaining oil in a non-stick frying pan, add, the garlic and mushrooms and cook for 2–3 minutes. Add the tomatoes and peas and cook for a further 2–3 minutes. Season with black pepper. Arrange the vegetables on 4 serving plates, top each with a duck breast and spoon over the warm vinaigrette. Serve with sauté potatoes.

4 PORTIONS: 352 KCALS, 43G PROTEIN, 15G FAT, 2.5G SATURATED FAT, 11G CARBOHYDRATE, 4.7G SUGAR, 3G FIBRE, 0.9G SALT, 354MG SODIUM

guinea fowl with apple, wild mushroom and tarragon

I made this recipe using chicken for dinner while visiting friends in the beautiful Vosges countryside of France. It went down well made with ingredients we had to hand in their kitchen and purchased at the wonderful local market that day in Gérardmer. There are some excellent wild mushroom varieties on the market, especially in autumn, and certain ones are available all year round.

1 tablespoon sunflower oil
4 x 180g skinless boneless guinea fowl breasts
freshly ground black pepper
200g mixed wild mushrooms (or button mushrooms), cleaned and sliced
½ garlic clove, crushed
100ml apple juice (no added sugar)

150ml chicken stock (see page 156; if using ready-made products or stock cubes use 'low-salt' varieties)
100ml semi-skimmed milk
1 tablespoon cornflour
1 teaspoon Dijon mustard
2 tablespoons chopped fresh tarragon

Serves 4

Heat a heavy-based frying pan with a squirt of oil-water spray. Season the guinea fowl breasts with black pepper, add to the pan and seal quickly on both sides without allowing to colour. Add the wild mushrooms and garlic and cook for a further 2–3 minutes.

Remove the guinea fowl and set aside. Add the apple juice and stock and cook for 2–3 minutes.

Whisk the milk and cornflour together and whisk into the stock. Simmer for 5 minutes. Add the mustard and tarragon, then return the guinea fowl to the sauce. Cook for a further 5-6 minutes until the fowl is tender and the sauce thick enough to coat the bird. Season with black pepper and serve.

4 PORTIONS: 244 KCALS, 39G PROTEIN, 5G FAT, 1.8G SATURATED FAT, 7G CARBOHYDRATE, 3.8G SUGAR, 0.4G FIBRE, 0.49G SALT, 193MG SODIUM

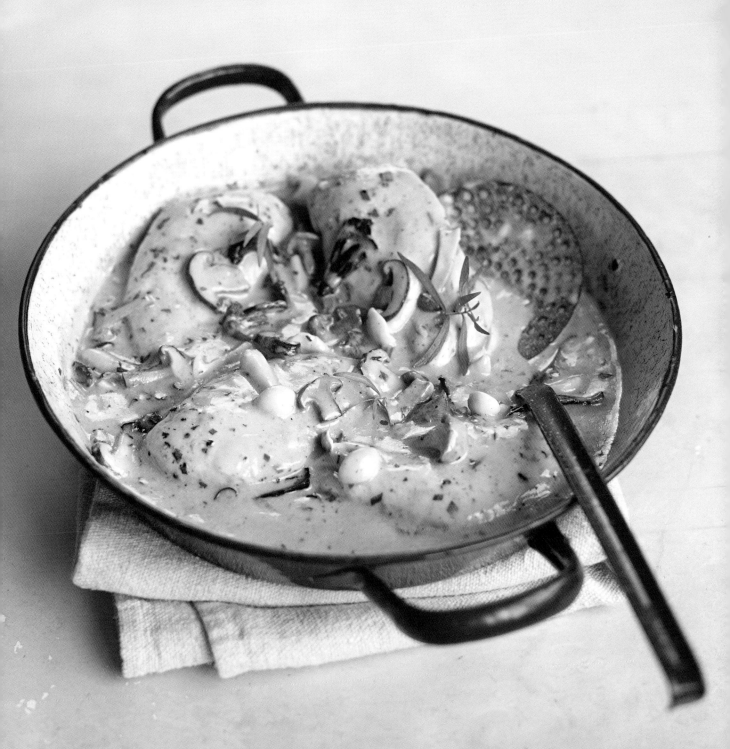

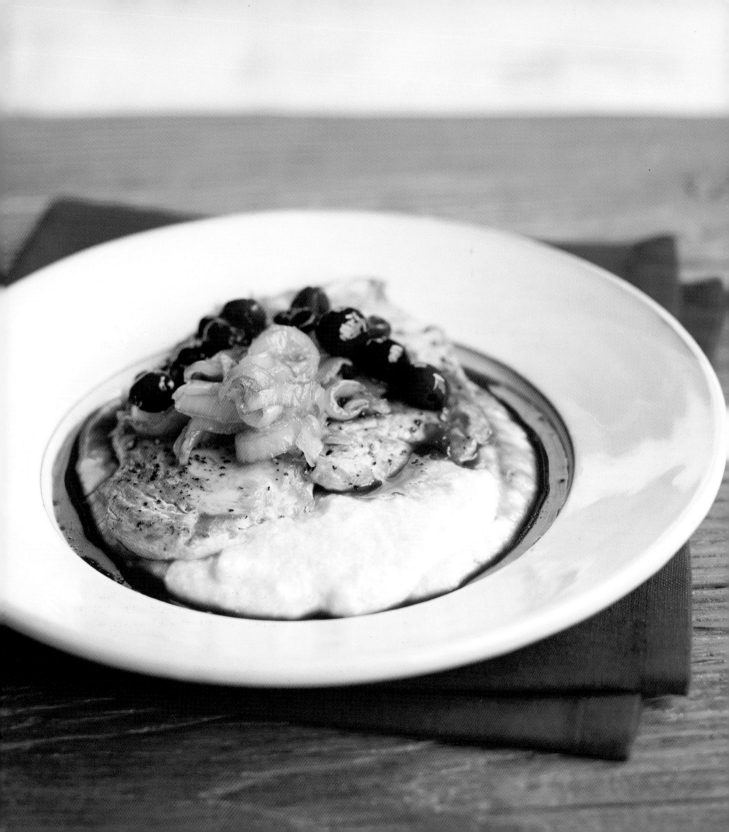

pheasant escalope with chicory and cranberries

Pheasants are available from October to February when the game season is really under way. They are generally sold as brace (two), but can also be purchased frozen. Game birds are very underrated in this country, I believe due to the fact that people are unsure how to cook them. In this recipe the pheasant breasts only are used, battered out into thin escalopes, making the cooking and timing much easier and reliable. Almond polenta makes a wonderful accompaniment but do check the label of quick-cook polenta as some brands contain added salt.

4 x 150g pheasant breasts, boneless, skin removed
4 Belgain endive (chicory), leaves separated, shredded coarsely
1 tablespoon maple syrup
2 tablespoons sunflower oil
1 tablespoon cider vinegar
150ml cranberry juice
1 tablespoon cranberry jelly (reduced-sugar if available)
150ml reduced chicken stock (see page 156; if using ready-made products or stock cubes use 'low-salt' varieties)
125g frozen cranberries
freshly ground black pepper

For the almond polenta
125g quick-cook polenta
50g ground almonds
1 small garlic clove, crushed
650ml semi-skimmed milk
few thyme sprigs

Serves 4

Place each pheasant breast between 2 sheets of clingfilm and, using a kitchen mallet or rolling pin, lightly batter them out to 2cm thick escalopes.

For the polenta, bring the milk, garlic and thyme to the boil, heat for 5 minutes, then remove the thyme. Slowly rain in the polenta and ground almonds in a stream, stirring constantly. Reduce the heat to the lowest setting, simmer the polenta for 8–10 minutes or until the polenta is cooked and the consistency of wet mashed potato. Keep warm.

Heat a non-stick pan, add the chicory, maple syrup and 500ml water and cook over a medium heat until the chicory is softened and caramelised. Remove from the heat and keep warm.

Heat the oil in a large non-stick frying pan, add the pheasant escalopes and cook over a high heat for 2–3 minutes on each side until pink and tender. Remove to a plate, cover with foil and keep warm.

Add the vinegar, cranberry juice, cranberry jelly and reduced stock to the pan and cook for 2–3 minutes. Strain through a fine sieve. Add the cranberries and cook for 4–5 minutes or until softened. Season with black pepper.

Place the polenta onto serving plates, top with the caramelised chicory and a pheasant escalope. Reheat the cranberry sauce for 2 minutes, then pour over the pheasant escalope and serve.

4 PORTIONS: 556 KCALS, 47.8G PROTEIN, 21.1G FAT, 4.6G SATURATED FAT, 44.2G CARBOHYDRATE, 19.8G SUGAR, 3.1G FIBRE, 0.34G SALT, 136MG SODIUM

turkey paillard with lentils and apricot vinaigrette

Turkey doesn't have to be roasted you know! Here the breast is sliced into escalopes, or paillards to use the more old-fashioned term, then grilled until succulent. Serve with earthy chestnuts and Puy lentils and a sweet apricot sauce. Steamed broccoli or spinach make a nice accompaniment.

2 tablespoons sunflower oil
1 onion, peeled and
  finely chopped
350g Puy lentils
4 x 200g escalopes of
  turkey breast
250g cooked frozen chestnuts
  (or vacuum packed)

For the vinaigrette
8 dried apricots, soaked in hot
  water until plump, drained,
  dried and chopped
1 tablespoon balsamic vinegar
½ teaspoon Dijon mustard
4 tablespoons olive oil
1 teaspoon chopped fresh
  rosemary
1 tablespoon honey
freshly ground black pepper

Serves 4

Heat the oil in a heavy-based pan, add the onion and cook until golden. Add the lentils and enough water to cover, then cook for 15–20 minutes or until just tender, but still retaining a bite. Drain well and keep warm. Toss through the chestnuts.

Make the vinaigrette by mixing all the ingredients in a bowl. Season to taste with black pepper.

Preheat a char grill or grill pan. When hot, season the turkey with black pepper and cook on the grill for 3–4 minutes each side until cooked through.

Add a little of the vinaigrette to the lentils, and spoon onto individual serving plates. Top each with a grilled turkey paillard, spoon over the remaining apricot vinaigrette and serve.

4 PORTIONS: 786 KCALS, 72.7G PROTEIN, 21.7G FAT, 3.2G SATURATED FAT, 79.9G CARBOHYDRATE, 19G SUGAR, 12.2G FIBRE, 0.37G SALT, 149MG SODIUM

zaatar-spiced chicken with arabic slaw

Zaatar is a Middle Eastern spice mix consisting of dried thyme, sesame seeds and sumac, a lemon-flavoured berry, which can be found in good delicatessens and stores. Zaatar can also be purchased ready-blended from Middle Eastern stores. Panko breadcrumbs are a dry and crispy breadcrumb used extensively in Japanese cooking. They add a wonderful crunch to fried foods and are well worth sourcing. Serve with some toasted wholemeal pitta breaded fingers.

1 tablespoon dried thyme
1 tablespoon sesame seeds
1 tablespoon sumac
1 tablespoon olive oil
100g panko breadcrumbs
freshly ground black pepper
650g chicken thighs, skinless and
  boneless, cut into 3cm cubes
2 eggs, beaten with 1 tablespoon
  water

For the slaw
1 red onion, peeled and
  thinly sliced
½ small cucumber,
  thinly sliced
1 red pepper, deseeded and
  thinly sliced
50g fresh mint leaves
50g fresh coriander leaves
juice of ½ lemon
2 tablespoons reduced-fat
  mayonnaise

Serves 4

In a dish, prepare the zaatar by mixing together the thyme, sesame seeds and sumac. Add the panko crumbs and a little black pepper.

Dip the chicken pieces in the beaten egg mixture until covered, then into the spice mix. Thread onto 4 metal or pre-soaked wooden skewers, 5–6 pieces per skewer.

Heat the olive oil in a large non-stick frying pan, add the skewers and fry over a medium heat for 8–10 minutes, turning often. Meanwhile, toss all the ingredients for the slaw in a bowl and season with a little black pepper.

Serve the skewers with a pile of the slaw alongside, and with hot toasted pitta fingers.

4 PORTIONS: 416 KCALS, 43G PROTEIN, 17G FAT, 4G SATURATED FAT, 24G CARBOHYDRATE, 4.6G SUGAR, 1.6G FIBRE, 0.87G SALT, 344MG SODIUM

spanish-style lamb stew

In Spain this typical lamb stew is known as 'Caldereta'; this is my adaption of the dish.

4 garlic cloves, crushed
2 bay leaves
1 teaspoon Spanish
  smoked paprika
freshly ground black pepper
300ml tomato purée
  (no added salt)
1 teaspoon caster sugar
2 tablespoons red wine vinegar
6 x 150g lamb neck fillets or
  rumps, trimmed of all visible fat

1 tablespoon olive oil
2 onions, finely chopped
2 green peppers, deseeded
  and cut into large pieces
1 head fennel, cut into large
  pieces
400g baby new potatoes
2 tablespoons chopped fresh
  flat-leaf parsley
1 tablespoon chopped fresh
  oregano

Serves 6

In a blender, place the garlic, bay leaves, smoked paprika, black pepper, tomato puree, sugar and vinegar with a little water and blitz to a paste.

Cut the lamb into large cubes, place in a dish then toss with the marinade. Cover with clingfilm and leave to marinate for 2 hours at room temperature.

Heat the olive oil in a heavy-based non-stick pan, add the onion, peppers and fennel and cook for 4–5 minutes until the vegetables are slightly softened. Add the marinated meat and juices to the pan, cover with water, bring to the boil, reduce the heat and simmer.

After 30 minutes, add the new potatoes, parsley and oregano and simmer in the sauce for a further 30 minutes or until cooked. Adjust the seasoning and serve.

4 PORTIONS: 437 KCALS, 34.1G PROTEIN, 23.4G FAT, 10.7G SATURATED FAT, 23.8G CARBOHYDRATE, 12.1G SUGAR, 4.1G FIBRE, 0.29G SALT, 116MG SODIUM

rump of lamb niçoise with aioli

A dish reminiscent of the colours and flavours of Provence.

1 aubergine, cut into large cubes
1 green courgette, thickly sliced
1 yellow courgette, thickly sliced
1 head fennel, cut into large cubes
1 red pepper, deseeded and cut into thick strips
1 yellow pepper, deseeded and cut into thick strips
8 garlic cloves, peeled
1 tablespoon roughly chopped fresh rosemary
2 tablespoons olive oil
freshly ground black pepper
4 x 150g lamb rumps, all excess fat removed

For the aioli
100ml reduced-fat mayonnaise
½ garlic clove, crushed
juice of ¼ lemon

Serves 4

Preheat the oven to 200°C/400°F/gas mark 6.

Toss the vegetables and rosemary in the olive oil, season with black pepper, place in a roasting tin and roast for 30–40 minutes until tender and lightly charred. Season the lamb with black pepper. After 20 minutes, place the lamb rumps on the vegetables and continue to roast until all ingredients are cooked.

For the aioli, mix all the ingredients together in a bowl and season with black pepper.

Divide the vegetables between 4 serving plates, carve each lamb rump into 4 slices and place on top of the vegetables. Drizzle aioli around the plate and serve.

4 PORTIONS: 410 KCALS, 34.4G PROTEIN, 25.5G FAT, 7.9G SATURATED FAT, 11.6G CARBOHYDRATE, 8.7G SUGAR, 4.6G FIBRE, 0.88G SALT, 350MG SODIUM

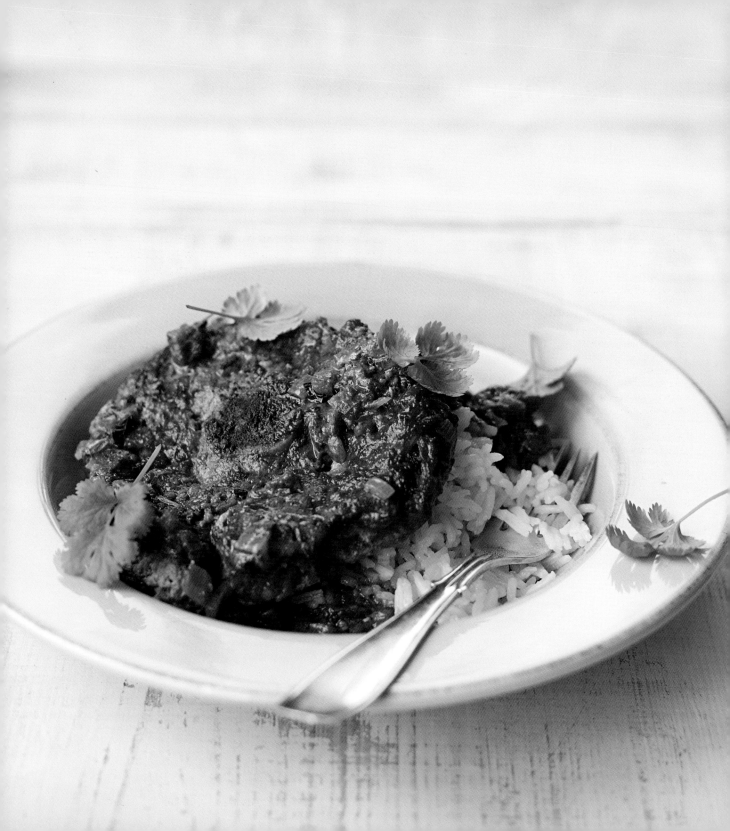

lamb osso bucco (indian style)

You may be confused by this dish. Classic Osso Bucco is traditionally an Italian dish made with veal shank, which is fairly expensive and often difficult to obtain. In this recipe I use lamb gigots, and flavour the sauce with wonderful Indian spices using the same method. A dish for hearty meat eaters, serve with saffron rice.

2 garlic cloves, crushed
10cm piece root ginger, peeled and chopped
100ml natural low-fat yogurt
4 x 250–275g lean gigot lamb steaks (leg steaks)
freshly ground black pepper
2 tablespoons sunflower oil
1 onion, peeled and chopped
1 red chilli, finely chopped
1 teaspoon curry powder
½ teaspoon ground turmeric
1 teaspoon ground cumin
1 teaspoon ground cardamom
400g can chopped tomatoes
1 tablespoon tomato purée
1 tablespoon brown sugar
1 litre chicken stock (see page 156; if using
   ready-made stock or cubes use 'low salt' varieties)
1 tablespoon chopped fresh mint
1 tablespoon chopped fresh coriander

Serves 4

Firstly place the garlic and ginger in a blender with the yogurt and blitz to a paste. Place the lamb steaks in a dish, season with black pepper then add the yogurt mixture, mix well together, cover with clingfilm and place in the fridge to marinate overnight.

Preheat the oven to 180°C/350°F/gas mark 4.

Heat the oil in a heavy-based flameproof casserole dish. When hot, remove the lamb from its marinade, wiping off any excess, add to the pan and fry until golden on both sides. Remove from the pan and set aside. Reserve the marinade.

Add the onion and chilli to the pan and cook gently until onions are lightly golden. Add the curry powder, turmeric, cumin and cardamom and cook for 1 minute. Add the marinade, tomatoes, tomato purée, sugar and stock and bring to the boil.

Return the lamb to the sauce, cover the casserole with a lid and place in the oven to braise for up to 1 hour until the lamb is tender. Adjust the seasoning of the sauce. Add the mint and coriander to garnish.

Place each lamb steak on a bed of saffron rice, then pour over the braising sauce and serve.

4 PORTIONS: 470 KCALS, 50.3G PROTEIN, 24.5G FAT, 9.7G SATURATED FAT, 13G CARBOHYDRATE, 9.5G SUGAR, 1.8G FIBRE, 0.68G SALT, 270MG SODIUM

mustard lamb with garlic and mint

To roast the garlic, simply break into cloves, place them in a pouch of foil with a spoonful of olive oil and bake at 180°C for up to 30 minutes until the garlic is soft and lightly caramelised. Leave to cool, then slip the cooked garlic cloves from their skins.

4 tablespoons olive oil
8 lamb cutlets, trimmed of
  excess fat
freshly ground black pepper
50ml dry white wine
300ml reduced chicken stock
  (see page 156; if using ready-
  made products or stock cubes
  use 'low-salt' varieties)
1 teaspoon Dijon mustard
1 tablespoon mint jelly
4 courgettes, cut into thick slices

For the garlic oil
3 tablespoons olive oil
12 roasted garlic cloves
  (see introduction)
2 tomatoes, blanched,
  skinned, deseeded and
  cut into small dice
juice of ½ lemon
1 tablespoon chopped
  fresh mint

Serves 4

Heat 2 tablespoons of the olive oil in a non-stick frying pan, season the lamb with black pepper and fry for 3–4 minutes on each side until pink (a little longer if you prefer them more well done). Remove from the pan and keep warm.

Add the wine and stock to the pan and boil for 5 minutes. Add the mustard and mint jelly and stir together to form a sauce.

In a separate pan, sauté the courgettes in the remaining oil for 4–5 minutes until golden and tender. Season with black pepper, remove and keep warm.

For the garlic oil, heat the olive oil, add the roasted garlic, tomatoes, lemon juice and mint and cook on the lowest heat for 2–3 minutes to infuse. Season with black pepper.

To serve arrange the lamb on a bed of courgettes, pour a little of the mustard mint sauce around, and a little roasted garlic oil over the lamb.

4 PORTIONS: 456 KCALS, 30.5G PROTEIN, 32.6G FAT, 9G SATURATED FAT, 9.7G CARBOHYDRATE, 7.3G SUGAR, 2.3G FIBRE, 0.34G SALT, 135MG SODIUM

pork chop with mixed summer beans and grilled peach

This is a lovely dish to make during the summer when peaches are available, and out of this world. Saying that, there are some good quality preserved or canned varieties on the market, which could be substituted. For the best results peel the peaches.

1 tablespoon sunflower oil
4 x 175g pork chops, all excess
  fat removed
1 tablespoon reduced-sugar
  peach jam
2 tablespoons balsamic vinegar
2 large peaches, halved and
  stoned

100ml dry sherry
100ml peach nectar
200ml reduced chicken stock
  (see page 156; if using
  ready-made products or stock
  cubes use 'low-salt' varieties)
250g yellow wax beans
300g French green beans
freshly ground black pepper

Serves 4

Heat a non-stick frying pan and add the oil. Season the pork chops with black pepper, add to the pan and cook on a medium heat for 4–5 minutes on each side until golden. Remove from the pan and keep warm.

Return the pan to the heat, add the peach jam and vinegar and cook for 30 seconds. Add the peach halves, cut-side down and lightly caramelise in the vinegar syrup. When slightly softened, remove and keep warm.

To the pan add the sherry, peach nectar and stock, reduce by half in volume, then strain through a sieve into a clean pan.

Cook the beans in separate pans of boiling water until tender, then drain and season with black pepper.

Arrange the beans on 4 individual serving plates and top each with a cooked pork chop. Place a caramelised peach on each chop, pour over the sauce and serve.

4 PORTIONS: 333 KCALS, 43G PROTEIN, 10G FAT, 2.2G SATURATED FAT, 16G CARBOHYDRATE, 14.6G SUGAR, 4.4G FIBRE, 0.31G SALT, 123MG SODIUM

lamb neck fillet with red cabbage caponata

A caponata is a sweet and sour relish, served as an accompaniment to fish or meat dishes. Traditionally made with aubergine and celery, this one to serve with the lamb is made with red cabbage following the same principles. Serve with cubes of roasted potatoes cooked with garlic and sage.

4 x 150g lamb neck fillets
2 tablespoons olive oil
freshly ground black pepper
1 tablespoon fresh thyme leaves
400ml reduced chicken stock

For the caponata
2 tablespoons sunflower oil

1 small red cabbage, very
 thinly sliced
1 red onion, thinly sliced
175ml red wine vinegar
4 tablespoons maple syrup
50g raisins,soaked in water for
 30 minutes, drained dried
2 tablespoons toasted pine nuts

Serves 4

Preheat the oven to 200°C/400°F/gas mark 6.

For the caponata, heat the oil in a heavy-based pan, add the onions and red cabbage, reduce the heat and cook, stirring occasionally, for about 20 minutes until the cabbage and onion have softened.

Add the vinegar and maple syrup and continue cooking until the vegetables are cooked and caramelised. Add the raisins and pine nuts and mix well. Remove from the heat and keep warm. Brush the lamb fillets all over with the olive oil and season with black pepper and thyme.

Heat a non-stick frying pan. When hot, add the lamb and seal, turning occasionally until golden all over. Place in the oven and cook for 10–12 minutes. Remove and keep warm. Add the stock to the pan juices, return to the boil and season with black pepper.

Cut the lamb into thick slices, dress on the cabbage, pour pan juices over the lamb and serve.

4 PORTIONS: 549 KCALS, 32.7G PROTEIN, 35.8G FAT, 12.3G SATURATED FAT, 25.5G CARBOHYDRATE, 22.0G SUGAR, 3.2G FIBRE, 0.35G SALT, 138MG SODIUM

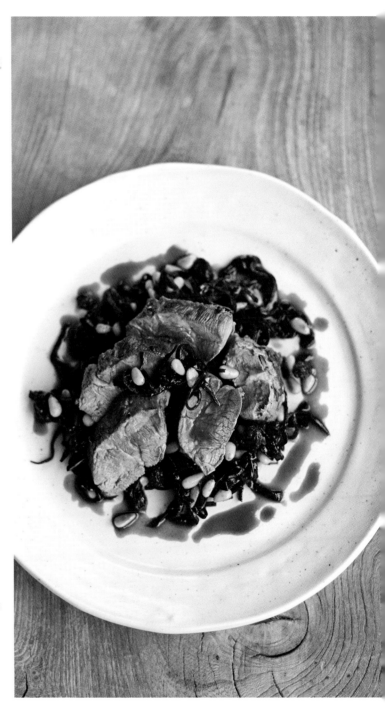

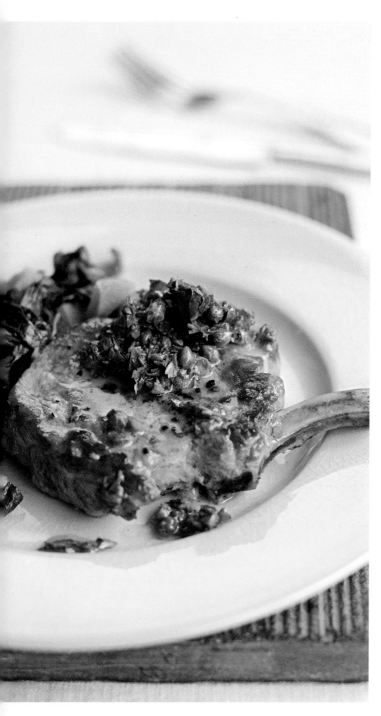

pork chop with chard, raisins and green sauce

It is vitally important not to overcook pork. I prefer to serve it when it is still a little pink but this is not advisable for pregnant women, young children or the elderly. However, adding a little water during the cooking process should help keep it moist and juicy.

4 x 175g pork chops, fat removed
freshly ground black pepper
8 large fresh Swiss chard leaves, roughly chopped
2 tablespoons olive oil
1 garlic clove, crushed
50g raisins, soaked in warm water, for 30 minutes, drained
50g ready-to-eat dried apricots, cut into pieces

For the green sauce
2 tablespoons chopped fresh flat-leaf parsley
2 tablespoons chopped fresh mint
½ teaspoon Dijon mustard
1 tablespoon capers, rinsed, drained and chopped
1 garlic clove, crushed
½ teaspoon sugar
3 tablespoons olive oil
1 tablespoon white wine vinegar

Serves 4

Quickly prepare the green sauce. Place the herbs, mustard, capers, garlic and sugar in a small blender, add the oil and vinegar and blitz to a coarse paste.

In a pan, heat half the olive oil and garlic together. Add the chard stems and season with a little pepper. Add 100ml water and cook for 5 minutes. Add the chard leaves, apricots and raisins and cook for a further 3–4 minutes until tender.

Meanwhile, heat a non-stick frying pan and add the remaining oil. Season the pork chops with the pepper, add to the pan and colour on both sides. Reduce the heat, add a spoonful of water, cover the pan and cook gently for 5–6 minutes until just cooked. Keep warm.

To serve, place the pork chops on serving plates, garnish with a spoonful of the green sauce and place the braised chard alongside. Serve immediately.

4 PORTIONS: 381 KCALS, 36.2G PROTEIN, 19.3G FAT, 3.6G SATURATED FAT, 16.8G CARBOHYDRATE, 14.5G SUGAR, 1.3G FIBRE, 0.90G SALT, 356MG SODIUM

pork schnitzel with apple, sage, celeriac remoulade

Schnitzel is the term for a German or Austrian meat preparation consisting of a batted out thin escalope of veal or pork in a crispy crumb crust. I like to serve it with mashed potato or small roasted new potatoes.

4 x 175g pork chops or loin, any bone and visible
    fat removed
1 egg, beaten
3 tablespoons semi-skimmed milk
75g dried wholemeal breadcrumbs
3 tablespoons sunflower oil
2 Granny Smith apples, cored and cut
    into 6 wedges
1 teaspoon brown sugar
250ml apple juice (no added sugar)
100ml reduced chicken stock (see page 156;
    if using ready-made stock or cubes use
    'low salt' varieties)
8 small sage leaves

For the celeriac remoulade
1 medium celeriac (approx 300g), peeled
juice of ½ lemon
2 teaspoons Dijon mustard
2 tablespoons reduced-fat mayonnaise
freshly ground black pepper

Serves 4

Using a kitchen mallet or large rolling pin, lightly flatten the pork chops between 2 sheets of clingfilm. Mix the egg and milk together in a bowl. Dip the pork escalopes in the egg mix then dredge them through the breadcrumbs, ensuring they are coated well all over.

To make the remoulade, grate the celeriac coarsely in a bowl, then add the lemon juice. Leave for 5 minutes, then squeeze out all the excess liquid in your hands. Dry in a cloth, then place in a bowl. Stir in the mustard and mayonnaise and season with black pepper.

Heat a non-stick frying pan with 1 tablespoon of the oil, add the apple wedges and cook for 1 minute until golden.

Sprinkle over the sugar and lightly caramelise in the pan. Add the apple juice, stock and sage and cook until the apples are tender and the sauce reduced by half in volume.

Heat another large non-stick pan with the remaining 2 tablespoons of oil, when hot add the schnitzel, cook for 2–3 minutes until golden and crispy.

Spoon the apples in the sauce onto serving plates, top each with a schnitzel, garnish with the celeriac remoulade and serve.

4 PORTIONS: 460 KCALS, 44G PROTEIN, 20.6G FAT, 4.4G SATURATED FAT, 26.1G CARBOHYDRATE, 16.4G SUGAR, 4.8G FIBRE, 1.05G SALT, 415MG SODIUM

beef fillet with sweet potato and hazelnut purée

This dish is an adaptation of a recipe by my good friend Dean Fearing, a pioneer of Southern cuisine in Texas during the nineties. Nutella is a popular chocolate and hazelnut spread, available in most supermarkets.

½ tablespoon maple syrup
1 tablespoon balsamic vinegar
1 teaspoon coarsely ground black pepper
½ teaspoon fresh thyme leaves
4 x 140g beef fillet steaks
2 large sweet potatoes
25g mono- or polyunsaturated spread
1 tablespoon Nutella (chocolate and hazelnut spread)
2 tablespoons sunflower oil
300g baby onions
1 teaspoon caster sugar
400ml reduced chicken stock (see page 156;
    if using ready-made products or stock cubes
    use 'low-salt' varieties)
200g mixed wild mushrooms, cleaned and trimmed

Serves 4

In a shallow dish, combine the maple syrup with the balsamic vinegar, black pepper and thyme. Add the beef fillets, mix well with the marinade, cover and leave in the fridge to marinate overnight.

Preheat the oven to 180°C/350°F/gas mark 4.

Prick the sweet potatoes all over with a small fork, place them on a sheet of foil, scrunch it up to seal up the foil, place on a baking sheet in the oven for 30 minutes until soft. Leave to cool slightly before peeling.

Pass the sweet potatoes through a sieve or mash until smooth, add the spread and Nutella, mix again and season well with black pepper. Keep warm.

Heat 1 tablespoon of oil in a non-stick frying pan, add the baby onions and fry until golden. Add the sugar and continue to cook until caramelised. Add the stock and simmer until tender. Add the wild mushrooms, cook for 2 minutes, and set aside.

Heat the remaining oil in a non-stick frying pan and cook the beef fillets until golden all over – 3–4 minutes on each side (for medium), longer if you prefer them more well done. Remove from the pan and keep warm. Add 2 tablespoons of the beef marinade to the pan, along with the reserved onion and mushroom mixture and heat gently.

Arrange the sweet potatoes on serving plates, top with beef, pour over the sauce and serve.

4 PORTIONS: 479 KCALS, 34.8G PROTEIN, 20.5G FAT, 5.4G SATURATED FAT, 41.4G CARBOHYDRATE, 16.2G SUGAR, 5G FIBRE, 0.55G SALT, 217MG SODIUM

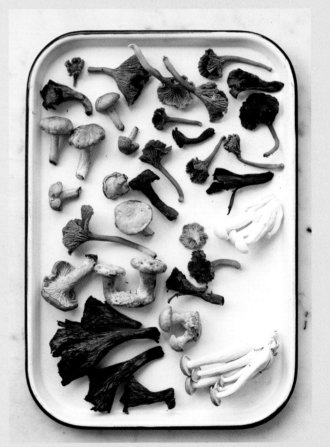

spice-grilled venison with beetroot and apple risotto

Venison is a nice lean choice of game. The spice crust adds a fragrant heat and works well with the slightly sweet-tasting risotto. Farmed venison is good and widely available, although wild venison does have a more intense flavour. I often serve this dish with a purée of broccoli.

8 x 80g lean venison medallions
½ teaspoon black peppercorns, lightly cracked
1 teaspoon fennel seeds, lightly cracked
2 tablespoons chopped fresh coriander
1 tablespoon chopped fresh mint
2.5cm piece root ginger, peeled and grated
1 tablespoon olive oil

For the risotto
700ml chicken stock (see page 156; if using
   ready-made products or stock cubes use
   'low-salt' varieties)
100ml red wine
juice of 1 small raw beetroot
2 tablespoons olive oil
1 small onion, chopped
1 large cooked beetroot, cut into small dice
250g risotto rice (e.g. Arborio, carnaroli)
½ Granny Smith apple, peeled and grated
knob of unsalted butter, to finish

Serves 4

Place the venison medallions in a shallow dish. In a bowl, mix together all the seasoning ingredients except the oil. Liberally season the venison all over with the spice mix, cover with clingfilm and leave to marinate at room temperature for 1 hour.

For the risotto, place the stock, wine and half the beetroot juice in a pan. Bring to the boil and simmer for 5 minutes.

Heat the oil in a heavy-based saucepan, add the onion and beetroot and cook gently for 2 minutes. Add the rice and stir to coat well with the beetroot.

Add the hot stock gradually, about 150ml at a time, ensuring it is completely evaporated before adding more, stirring all the time. This will take up to 20–25 minutes in all, by which time the rice should be just tender but while retaining a little bite (al dente).

Add the grated apple along with the remaining beetroot juice and butter to finish, which will give it added richness. Season with a little black pepper.

While the risotto is cooking, cook your venison. Heat a chargrill or grill pan until hot, brush the venison medallions liberally with a little oil and cook on the hot grill for 3–4 minutes each side for pink or longer if you prefer your meat more well done.

Spoon the beetroot risotto onto serving plates, top with the spiced venison medallions and serve.

4 PORTIONS: 505 KCALS, 42G PROTEIN, 13G FAT, 2.7G SATURATED FAT, 56G CARBOHYDRATE, 5.2G SUGAR, 2G FIBRE, 0.37G SALT, 145MG SODIUM

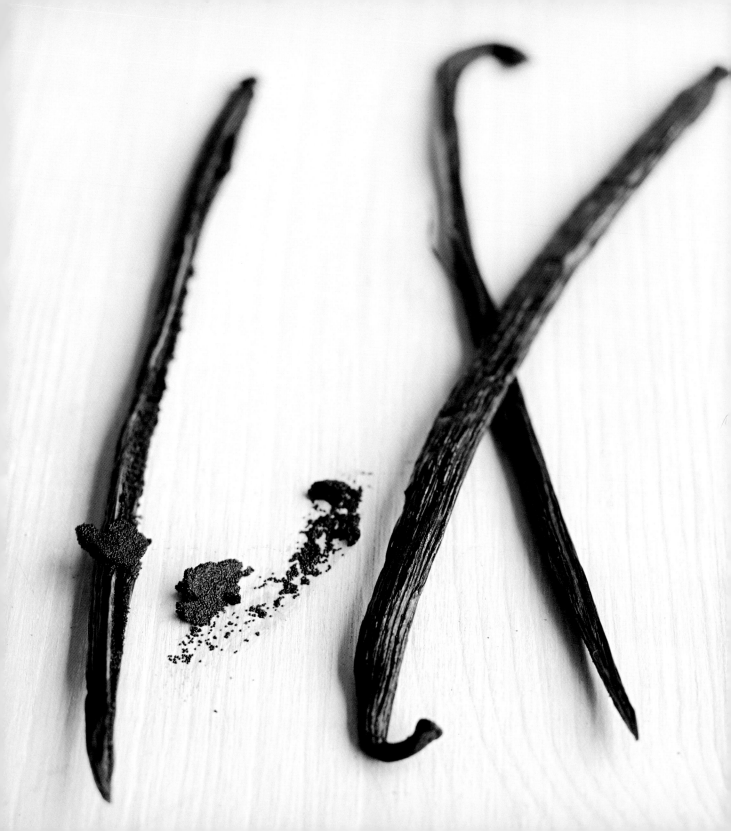

chapter five
desserts

almond milk custard with saffron and rosewater

Smooth, silky custards flavoured with saffron and rosewater are inspired by the Middle East. Garnish with some juicy raspberries or wild strawberries for an extra treat.

50g whole blanched almonds, toasted	2 tablespoons custard powder
350ml semi-skimmed milk	2 tablespoons rosewater
40g caster sugar	1 tablespoons Amaretto liquor (optional)
½ teaspoon vanilla extract	fresh berries and toasted flaked almonds, to serve
good pinch of saffron	icing sugar, to dust
2 eggs, plus 2 egg yolks	

Serves 4

Place the whole almonds in a blender and blitz until finely ground. Bring the milk, half the sugar and the vanilla extract to the boil in a pan. Remove from the heat, add the ground almonds and saffron and leave to infuse for 15 minutes.

In a bowl, whisk together the eggs, egg yolks and remaining sugar until light and fluffy, then whisk in the custard powder. Whisk in the almond milk, rosewater and Amaretto, if using.

Clean the saucepan and return the custard to it. Heat gently, stirring all the time, until it thickens (do not allow to boil). Pour the custard into individual gratin-style dishes or ramekins. Place on a tray and transfer to the fridge for up to 2 hours or until firmly set.

To serve, top with the chosen berries and flaked almonds and dust liberally with icing sugar.

4 PORTIONS: 260 KCALS, 11G PROTEIN, 15G FAT, 3.3G SATURATED FAT, 20G CARBOHYDRATE, 15.5G SUGAR, 0.9G FIBRE, 0.26G SALT, 104MG SODIUM

bananas 'en papillote' with banana sorbet

Opening these baked paper parcels at the table and releasing the aroma of the sweet fragrant spices adds a little theatre to the dessert. Bananas are a good source of potassium, which can help lower blood pressure; apricots and orange juice also provide potassium.

400g fresh apricots, stoned and chopped	4 small cinnamon sticks
150ml orange juice (fresh or pre-packed)	8 star anise pods
1 tablespoon caster sugar	4 medium ripe bananas
2 vanilla pods, split lengthways	banana sorbet, to serve (see page 148)
	few small mint laves, to garnish

Serves 4

Preheat the oven to 200°C/400°F/gas mark 6.

Place the apricots, orange juice and sugar in a pan, add the vanilla, cinnamon and star anise pods and cook gently for 10 minutes, until the apricots are very soft. Remove the spices and set aside.

Transfer the apricots to a blender and blitz until very smooth.

Cut 4 pieces of aluminium foil each 25x15cm and lay on a work surface. Place one peeled banana on each piece and fold up the sides of the foil into a neat boat shape.

Pour the apricot sauce over the bananas and tuck in the reserved spices (vanilla, anise pods and cinnamon). Fold up the edges of each parcel and seal it by scrunching it up at the top. Place on a baking sheet and bake for 15–20 minutes.

Serve the parcels to your guests at the table. When opened, place a ball of banana sorbet alongside and scatter with mint.

4 PORTIONS: 156 KCALS, 2G PROTEIN, 1G FAT, 0.1G SATURATED FAT, 38G CARBOHYDRATE, 34.9G SUGAR, 2.7G FIBRE, 0.02G SALT, 7MG SODIUM

grilled fruit kebabs in balsamic vinegar syrup

A simple and delicious dessert. You can vary the fruits according to the season and to your personal preference but remember the fruits chosen must be firm enough to withstand the grilling process and not too ripe. The kebabs can be prepared in advance, then just cooked in the syrup when needed, though fruit cut and left to stand ahead of time loses a lot of its vitamin C content. The wooden skewers should be soaked for 1 hour in water prior to use: this stops them being charred and black when grilling, especially when using on a hot charcoal grill.

2 nectarines
4 red plums
zest and juice of 1 orange
225g pineapple, cut into bite-sized chunks
   (prepared weight)
2 bananas
12 large strawberries, halved
2 tablespoons Grand Marnier or other
   orange liqueur (optional)

For the syrup
2 tablespoons brown sugar
75ml balsamic vinegar

Serves 4

Cut the nectarines and plums in half, remove the centre stones, then cut each half into bite-sized chunks. Peel the bananas and cut into 3cm thick slices.

Place the orange juice and zest and liqueur, if using, in a bowl, add all the fruit pieces and toss together. Leave for 30 minutes.

Thread the marinated fruit pieces onto prepared wooden sticks, alternating colours for added visual appeal, allowing 2 kebabs per person. Refrigerate until needed.

To serve, preheat grill to its highest setting. Heat the sugar and vinegar together in a small saucepan for 3–4 minutes or until it becomes syrupy. Place the skewers on a grill pan, brush liberally with the syrup, then place under the grill to glaze for about 4–5 minutes, turning them regularly. Drizzle over any excess syrup and serve.

4 PORTIONS: 176 KCALS, 2.6G PROTEIN, 0.4G FAT, 0.1G SATURATED FAT, 42.9G CARBOHYDRATE, 41.8G SUGAR, 3.4G FIBRE, 0.02G SALT, 10MG SODIUM

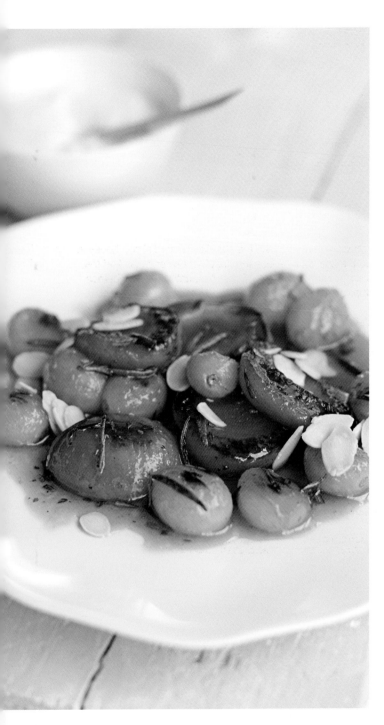

caramelised apricots with grapes and rosemary honey

For the purist who craves perfection, peeling the grapes with a small sharp knife lets them absorb the flavours of the juices in the pan. Whatever you decide it will be delicious! I have rarely used butter in this book, but here a little knob of good unsalted butter is essential.

12 fresh apricots, not too ripe (canned 'in juice' is fine)
300g seedless white grapes, peeled (unpeeled are fine)
2 tablespoons honey
small knob of unsalted butter
1 tablespoon brandy
1 teaspoon rosemary leaves, coarsely chopped
juice of 1 lemon

2 tablespoons flaked almonds, lightly toasted, to serve
low-fat natural yogurt, to serve

Serves 4

Halve the apricots and remove the centre stones.

Heat a large non-stick frying pan, add the apricots and grapes, then the honey and the butter and quickly caramelise over a high heat until golden.

Add the brandy and cook for 30 seconds, then add 4 tablespoons water. Add the rosemary and lemon juice and toss to form a sauce around the fruit.

Divide the fruit between 4 serving plates, scatter over the toasted almonds and serve with the yogurt.

4 PORTIONS: 130 KCALS, 2G PROTEIN, 1G FAT, 0.7G SATURATED FAT, 28G CARBOHYDRATE, 27.7G SUGAR, 2.3G FIBRE, 0.01G SALT, 5MG SODIUM

fromage frais with gooseberries and elderflower

This is one of the simplest yet tastiest dishes I know. The fromage frais is lightened to the texture of silky snow and topped with a fragrant and delicious honey-flavoured gooseberry compôte flavoured with elderflower. Gooseberries, to my sadness, have a very short early summer season, so use them at any opportunity to make wonderful sauces, tarts, puddings and compôtes. This dish is also great served for breakfast.

2 gelatine leaves
zest of ½ lemon
300ml low-fat fromage frais
1 tablespoon elderflower cordial
1 egg white
25g caster sugar

For the gooseberry compote
2 tablespoons elderflower cordial
75ml honey
225g gooseberries, not too ripe
1 teaspoon lemon juice

Serves 4

For the gooseberry compôte, place the elderflower cordial and honey in a pan, bring to the boil, then reduce the heat to a low simmer. Add the gooseberries and cook gently for 8–10 minutes, until the gooseberries are soft and the liquid is syrupy. Leave to cool and add lemon juice.

Place the gelatine leaves in a bowl, just cover with cold water and leave for 4–5 minutes to soften. Meanwhile, heat the elderflower cordial in a small pan. Squeeze out the gelatine and stir into the warmed cordial to melt, then leave to cool slightly.

Place the fromage frais and lemon zest in a bowl, pour over the cordial and gelatine liquid and mix well.

Whisk the egg white until stiff with half the sugar, then fold in the remaining sugar. Fold the whisked egg white gently into the fromage frais, ensuring it is well amalgamated. Divide the mixture between 4 serving bowls or glasses and place in the fridge to set for up to 1 hour.

Top each fromage frais with some gooseberry compôte and serve.

4 PORTIONS: 165 KCALS, 10G PROTEIN, 0G FAT, 0G SATURATED FAT, 33G CARBOHYDRATE, 32.6G SUGAR, 1.4G FIBRE, 0.15G SALT, 60MG SODIUM

citrus fruit float

This dessert takes me back to my childhood days, enjoying Mum's simple ice cream floats made by topping creamy vanilla ice cream with Coca Cola. In my more exotic version I combine a melange of colourful citrus fruits and an exotic lychee-based sorbet. You will find canned lychees work best for this sorbet and, of course, they are more readily available in stores.

For the sorbet
2 tablespoons caster sugar
100ml water
1 x 425g canned lychees in syrup
100ml pink grapefruit juice (preferably fresh with no added sugar)
2 tablespoons white rum (optional)

For the float
1 sweet orange
1 pink grapefruit
1 lime
1 piece stem ginger, finely chopped, plus 60ml syrup from the jar
2 sticks lemongrass, outer leaves removed, tender inner core finely chopped
300ml cream soda

Serves 4

For the sorbet, place the sugar and water in a pan. Slowly bring to the boil, simmer for 5 minutes until the sugar has dissolved. Remove from the heat and leave to cool.

Drain the lychees, reserving 150ml of their syrup. Purée the lychees in a blender, add the reserved lychee syrup, the cooled sugar syrup and the grapefruit juice and blitz to a smooth purée. Stir in the rum, if using.

Strain through a fine sieve, then transfer to an ice cream machine and freeze according to the manufacturer's instructions. Freeze if not using immediately.

For the float, cut away the peel and pith from all the citrus fruits, then segment the orange and grapefruit. Set aside.

In a small pan, gently heat the stem ginger and its syrup along with the lemongrass and mint for about 1 minute. Strain and set aside to cool.

To serve, place 1 or 2 scoops of the prepared lychee sorbet in a suitable martini or tumbler-style glass. Top with the fruit and drizzle over the cooled ginger syrup. Finally, pour over the soda and serve immediately while it is still bubbling.

4 PORTIONS: 227 KCALS, 1.5G PROTEIN, 0.2G FAT, 0G SATURATED FAT, 58.3G CARBOHYDRATE, 57.6G SUGAR, 2G FIBRE, 0.05G SALT, 23MG SODIUM

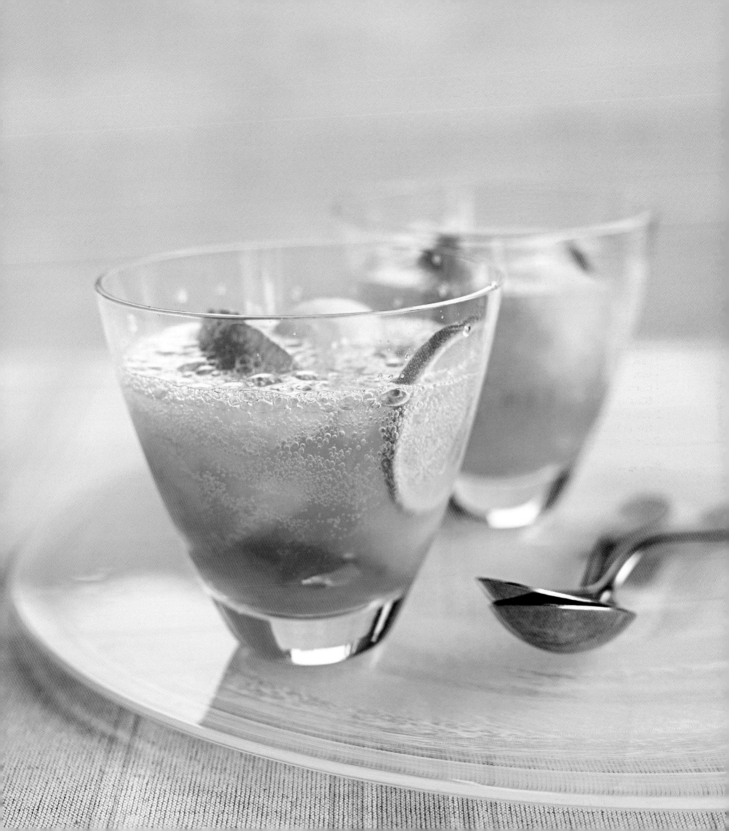

lemon verbena and berry gratin

Lemon verbena is a wonderful plant: by no means attractive or showy, it imports a fantastic lemony flavour to all manner of dishes from poultry to puddings, salad dressings, sorbets and ice creams.

200g raspberries
100g blackberries
100g blueberries
4 lemon verbena leaves, shredded
1 tablespoon kirsch liqueur (optional)
2 large eggs, separated
60g caster sugar
juice and zest of 2 lemons
1 teaspoon cornflour
a little icing sugar, to glaze

Serves 4

Preheat the oven to 180°C/350°F/gas mark 4.

Mix the berries together in a bowl, add the shredded verbena leaves and the kirsch, if using, and cover with clingfilm. Leave to steep for 20–30 minutes.

Meanwhile, beat the egg yolks and 50g of the sugar in a bowl until light and creamy. Stir in the lemon juice and zest and add the cornflour. Transfer to a heavy-based saucepan and heat, stirring, until it almost reaches boiling point and thickens (do not allow to boil). Leave to cool, stirring occasionally so no skin forms on the surface.

Whisk the egg whites with the remaining sugar until very stiff, then gently fold into the lemon sauce.

Divide the berries between 4 shallow ovenproof dishes and pour over the lemon sauce. Bake for 18–20 minutes or until puffed up and golden. Dust liberally with icing sugar and serve.

4 PORTIONS: 141 KCALS, 5G PROTEIN, 4G FAT, 0.9G SATURATED FAT, 24G CARBOHYDRATE, 22.7G SUGAR, 2.5G FIBRE, 0.12G SALT, 47MG SODIUM

hot cherries with red wine, liquorice and yogurt sorbet

I look forward to the arrival of the first summer cherries with great excitement and all manner of dishes are conjured up in my mind. Here is one of my favourites. People with very high blood pressure, though, should avoid eating too much liquorice as it can cause a rise in blood pressure. If in doubt, check with your doctor.

350g ripe cherries, stoned
zest of ½ lemon 2 tablespoons honey
100ml red wine
1 tablespoon reduced-sugar redcurrant jelly
½ tablespoon liquorice essence (or 2 liquorice sticks, peeled and chopped)
1 tablespoon chopped pistachio nuts, to serve (optional)

For the sorbet
400g low-fat yogurt
100ml semi-skimmed milk
50g caster sugar

Serves 4

For the sorbet, mix the yogurt, milk and sugar in a bowl, then transfer to an ice-cream maker and freeze following the manufacturer's instructions.

Place the zest, honey, red wine, redcurrant jelly and liquorice essence in a small pan and bring to the boil. Simmer for 2–3 minutes, then add the cherries. Simmer gently uncovered for 5 minutes until the cherries are tender and the cooking liquid has become syrupy.

Divide between 4 individual serving bowls and top with the yogurt sorbet. Sprinkle over the chopped pistachios if using. Serve immediately.

4 PORTIONS: 197 KCALS, 6.8G PROTEIN, 1.5G FAT, 0.9G SATURATED FAT, 39.5G CARBOHYDRATE, 39.2G SUGAR, 0.8G FIBRE, 0.23G SALT, 91MG SODIUM

italian mess
(an italian version)

Here's a play on the classic British dessert Eton Mess, usually comprising crushed fluffy meringue, soft raspberries and cream. In my version I take the flavours further afield while retaining the original concept. I think you will enjoy it.

4 large ripe peaches
4 small ready-made meringue nests
300ml low-fat fromage frais
4 amaretti biscuits, crushed
1 tablespoon Amaretto liqueur (optional)
cocoa powder, for dusting

Serves 4

Place the peaches in a bowl, cover with boiling water for 1 minute, then remove with a slotted spoon. Peel and cut the peaches in half, remove centre stones, then cut into large cubes and set aside.

In a bowl, crush the meringue into large pieces, add the fromage frais, crushed amaretti biscuits and liqueur, if using. Add two-thirds of the peaches and gently fold together.

Spoon the mixture into 4 individual tumbler-style glasses. Top with the remaining peaches and dust lightly with a little cocoa powder to serve.

4 PORTIONS: 176 KCALS, 8G PROTEIN, 1G FAT, 0.4G SATURATED FAT, 35G CARBOHYDRATE, 31G SUGAR, 2.5G FIBRE, 0.19G SALT, 75MG SODIUM

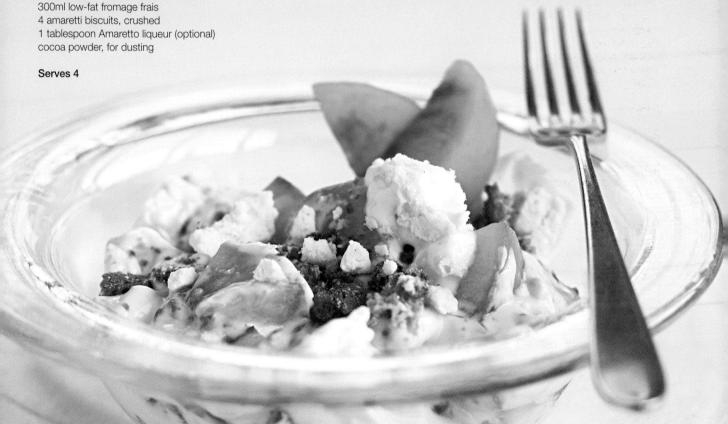

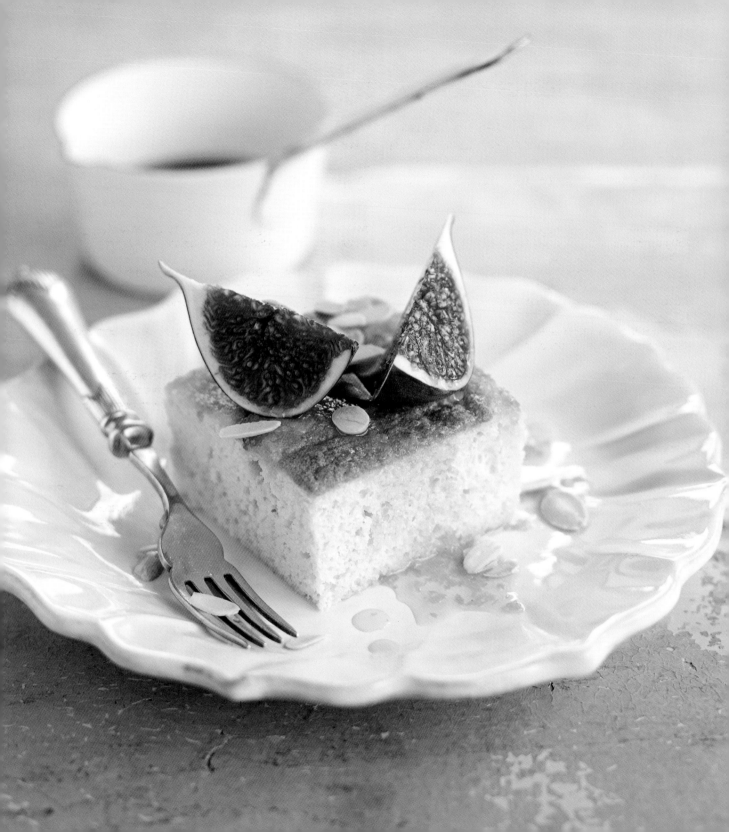

lemon polenta cake with figs

Polenta (or cornmeal) is often used in desserts in Italy and works
extremely well. Some brands, however, contain salt, so check the
label. The tanginess of the lemon syrup with figs brings the whole
thing together wonderfully well. Poached pears or kumquat orange
would be also very good.

6 eggs, separated
150g caster sugar
200ml low-fat natural yogurt
zest and juice of 2 lemons
90g polenta (ground cornmeal)
1 teaspoon low sodium baking powder
150g ground almonds
4 firm ripe figs, cut into quarters
2 tablespoons flaked almonds, lightly toasted

For the lemon syrup
4 lemons
2 tablespoons maple syrup
100ml water

Serves 8

Preheat the oven to 180°C/350°F/gas mark 4. Lightly grease an 18cm
cake tin, square or round and line the base with greaseproof paper.

To make the cake, beat the egg yolks in a bowl, add the sugar and whisk
until light, thick and creamy. Add the yogurt, lemon juice and zest. Using
a metal spoon, fold in the polenta, baking powder and ground almonds.

In a separate bowl, whisk the egg whites until stiff, then carefully fold into
the yogurt mix (do not overmix).

Spoon the mix into the prepared cake tin, smooth and level off the
surface. Bake for 30–40 minutes until golden and the cake is cooked
through when tested with the point of a small knife. Allow to cool slightly
before turning out onto a cooling rack.

For the syrup, zest 2 of the lemons and squeeze the juice from all 4.
Combine this with the syrup and water in a small pan and simmer for
2–3 minutes.

Cut the cake into squares or slices, top each with 2 half figs, drizzle over
the warm lemon syrup and scatter over the toasted almonds. Serve.

4 PORTIONS: 348 KCALS, 12.9G PROTEIN, 17.6G FAT, 2.5G SATURATED FAT,
36.7G CARBOHYDRATE, 28.1G SUGAR, 2.3G FIBRE, 0.29G SALT, 117MG SODIUM

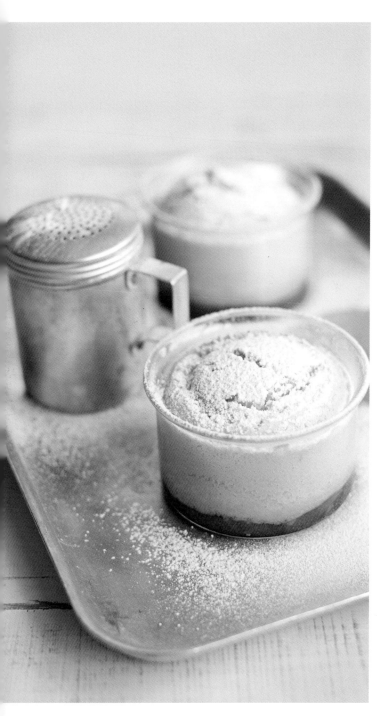

orange marmalade pudding

If you're a pudding lover like me you won't be disappointed with this recipe. The yogurt keeps it extremely light while the marmalade, which cooks in the bottom of the dish, adds a touch of bitterness, but a wonderful overall balance.

50g polyunsaturated spread
100g low-fat natural yogurt
75g caster sugar
1 teaspoon finely grated orange zest
2 eggs
75g plain flour
40g cornflour

1 teaspoon low sodium baking powder
100ml maple syrup
4 tablespoons reduced-sugar rough cut orange marmalade
icing sugar, to dust
low-fat natural yogurt or low-fat vanilla ice cream, to serve

Serves 6

Preheat the oven to 180°C/350°F/gas mark 4.

Lightly grease the insides of 6 individual soufflé or ramekin dishes (180ml). In a bowl, beat together the spread, yogurt, sugar and zest until light and fluffy. Beat in the eggs one at a time. Sift together the flour, cornflour and baking powder, then fold into the mixture.

Mix the maple syrup and marmalade together in a bowl, then divide the mix into the bases of the prepared dishes. Carefully spoon the pudding mix over the marmalade and fill them up to the top of each dish.

Cover the dishes with clingfilm and place in a deep baking tin. Pour enough boiling water into the pan to cover halfway up the sides of the pudding dishes.

Cover the pan, return to the boil, then reduce the heat to a simmer. Cook for 25–30 minutes or until a small knife inserted in the centre of a pudding comes out clean. Carefully remove the puddings and allow to cool slightly. Dust liberally with icing sugar and serve warm with low-fat yogurt or vanilla ice cream.

4 PORTIONS: 270 KCALS, 5G PROTEIN, 8G FAT, 1.9G SATURATED FAT, 47G CARBOHYDRATE, 29.6G SUGAR, 0.5G FIBRE, 0.39G SALT, 153MG SODIUM

summer fruit piperade

A piperade is a typical savoury dish from the Basque region made of peppers, onions and tomatoes cooked in olive oil and mixed with eggs – apparently the colours represent the Basque flag. In this sweet version I use fruit instead of vegetables, it makes an unusual dessert and is one that can be produced quickly.

1 teaspoon unsalted butter
2 tablespoons caster sugar
125g blackberries
150g raspberries
100g blueberries
6 eggs
1 small vanilla pod, split, seeds removed
   (or ½ teaspoon vanilla extract)
1 tablespoon kirsch (cherry liqueur)
2 tablespoons lightly toasted flaked almonds
icing sugar, to dust
low-fat fromage frais, to serve

Serves 4

Preheat the grill to its highest setting. Heat the butter in a medium-sized non-stick frying pan. Add 1 teaspoon of the sugar and the fruits and toss together in the pan for 1 minute.

In a bowl beat the eggs with the remaining sugar, vanilla seeds or extract and kirsch, if using. Pour the eggs over the fruit and stir gently with a fork as if making an omelette, until eggs are lightly set.

Sprinkle over the flaked almonds, dust liberally all over with icing sugar, then place under the grill until the sugar is lightly caramelised and golden. Carefully slip the omelette out of the pan onto a large serving plate and dust with more sugar. Serve with low-fat fromage blanc.

4 PORTIONS: 288 KCALS, 13G PROTEIN, 14G FAT, 3.6G SATURATED FAT, 26G CARBOHYDRATE, 26.2G SUGAR, 2.7G FIBRE, 0.33G SALT, 131MG SODIUM

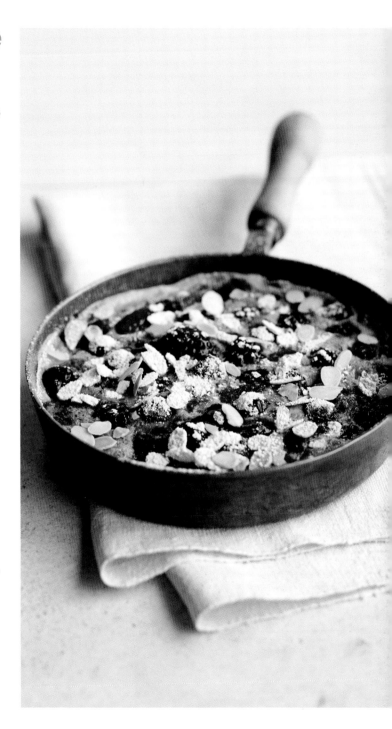

strawberry and watermelon jelly with sweet pesto

I love the freshness of this dessert, which should ideally only be made in the height of our summer when our strawberries are sweet juicy and utterly moreish.

500g ripe but firm strawberries,
　　hulled and halved
300g watermelon, skin removed
　　and cut into cubes
40g caster sugar
4 gelatine leaves
100ml rosé wine (or champagne!)

Serves 4

Place 300g of the strawberries and half the watermelon in a bowl and cover with the sugar and 200ml of water. Place the bowl above a pan of simmering water and leave to cook for 1½ hours, by which time the strawberries will have released their natural juices.

Remove the bowl and strain the juices through a fine sieve (or coffee filter) to give a clear sweet juice. Soak the gelatine leaves in a bowl of cold water for 4–5 minutes to soften. Measure 200ml of the juice and heat gently in a pan. Squeeze the gelatine leaves out in your hand, add to the juice and stir well until melted. Add the wine and transfer to a bowl to cool slightly.

Meanwhile, place the remaining strawberries and watermelon in shallow soup-style serving bowls or glasses. Top with the juice and place in fridge for about 30 minutes to set.

For the sweet pesto, place all the ingredients in a blender and whizz to a coarse texture. Top the jellies with a dollop of fromage frais, drizzle over the sweet pesto and serve.

4 PORTIONS: 204 KCALS, 8G PROTEIN, 3G FAT, 0.2G SATURATED FAT, 35G CARBOHYDRATE, 33.3G SUGAR, 1.8G FIBRE, 0.08G SALT, 32MG SODIUM

pear, rhubarb and cranberry crumble

A melange of sweet and sour-tasting fruits that combine together wonderfully, topped with a crisp oatmeal crust. Crumbles are so diverse and, let's face it, are loved by all. Other variations could be the addition of a little chopped candied ginger to the fruits or a blend of mixed nuts added to the crust. Why not create your own!

3 ripe firm pears, peeled and cored
475g rhubarb, trimmed and cut into 2.5cm lengths
50g brown sugar
zest of 1 orange
300g fresh (or frozen) cranberries
150ml cranberry juice

For the crumble
75g wholemeal flour
50g porridge oats
50g brown sugar
50g ground hazelnuts
50g polyunsaturated spread, warmed

Serves 4

Preheat oven to 200°C/400°F/gas mark 6.

Chop the pears into large pieces and place in a shallow ovenproof dish. Add the rhubarb, sugar, orange zest and cranberries and pour over the cranberry juice. Bake for 10 minutes.

Meanwhile, make the crumble. In a bowl combine the flour, oats, sugar and hazelnuts. Rub in the spread until it resembles breadcrumbs in texture. Remove the fruit from the oven and sprinkle over the crumble mix, pressing down lightly onto the fruit.

Bake for 25 minutes until bubbling and golden. Serve with low-fat yogurt or low-fat fromage frais.

4 PORTIONS: 447 KCALS, 8G PROTEIN, 18G FAT, 2.6G SATURATED FAT, 67G CARBOHYDRATE, 46.7G SUGAR, 9.8G FIBRE, 0.31G SALT, 122MG SODIUM

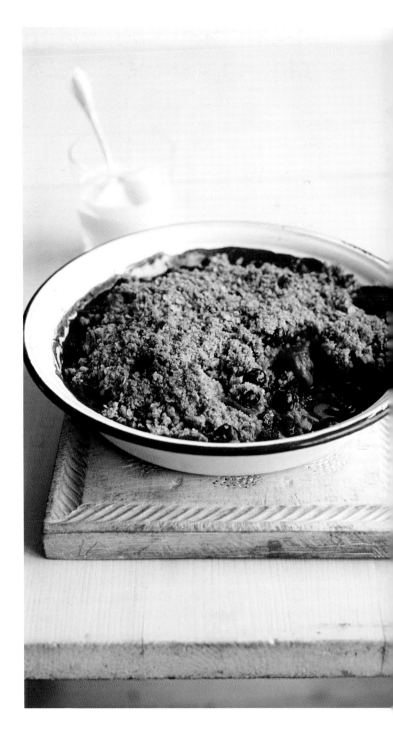

pecan bread pudding with banana sorbet

When I was a child growing up, bread pudding was a regular treat my mother made, a great way to use up any stale bread left over, though there wasn't much with three children! I thought it was time to return to it the full flavour, to rival the more popular bread and butter pudding! I have added a little decadence with the addition of chopped pecans, but they could be left out in favour of tradition and a much healthier option – maybe save the nuts for a special occasion. This sorbet is simply made in the freezer and does not require an ice cream machine.

225g wholemeal bread, ideally stale
100g mixed dried fruits (currants, raisins or sultanas)
50g soft brown sugar
50g suet
1 teaspoon mixed spice
1 large egg, beaten
a little semi-skimmed milk
300g pecan nuts, lightly crushed (optional)
icing sugar, to taste

For the sorbet
200g caster sugar
250ml Evian water
200g ripe banana, chopped
juice of ½ lemon

Serves 6

First make the sorbet. Place the sugar and water in a large pan and bring to the boil slowly to dissolve the sugar properly. Remove from the heat and allow to cool.

When cool, add the banana and lemon juice, transfer to a suitable freezer container and freeze for about 3 hours, until set around the edges.

Transfer the sorbet to a small blender and whizz until smooth. Return to the freezer until gently set; this will take 2–2 ½ hours. It is then ready for use.

Preheat the oven to 170°C/325°F/gas mark 3.

Cut or tear the bread into small chunks and place in a bowl. Add a little water just to cover and leave to soak for 45 minutes. Squeeze out the bread as dry as possible in your hands. Place in a bowl, add fruits, suet, sugar and spice and mix well. Add the egg and enough milk to bring mix to a drop consistency from a spoon.

Sprinkle the pecan nuts over the base of a lightly greased baking tin and carefully pour over the bread mixture. Bake for 1–1¼ hours until browned – it should be slightly firm to the touch. Leave to cool slightly before removing from the tin.

Cut into small squares, dust with icing sugar and serve with the Banana sorbet.

6 PORTIONS: 415 KCALS, 5.8G PROTEIN, 9.7G FAT, 0.6G SATURATED FAT, 81.3G CARBOHYDRATE, 64.7G SUGAR, 2.7G FIBRE, 0.30G SALT, 119MG SODIUM

pineapple and raisin clafoutis with curry ice cream

Traditional French clafoutis is made with sweet cherries, which is wonderful – the French often like it for a sweet breakfast treat. Any fruit can be used; here I use pineapple, which is available ready-prepared in many good supermarkets. The curry ice cream works wonderfully with the hot pudding: don't be put off by the thought of it on first reflection, it's a real dinner party talking point.

3 large eggs
40g caster sugar
1 tablespoon cornflour
2 tablespoons custard powder
400ml semi-skimmed milk
1 tablespoon ground almonds
100g raisins, soaked in warm water for
   30 minutes, drained and dried
225g ready-prepared fresh pineapple,
   cut into large chunks

for the ice cream
300ml semi-skimmed milk
1 teaspoon mild curry powder
4 egg yolks
100g caster sugar

Serves 4

First make the ice cream. Bring the milk and curry powder to the boil in a saucepan, then remove from the heat and leave to cool slightly. In a large bowl, whisk the egg yolks and sugar until light, fluffy and doubled in volume. Pour on the cooled milk, whisking all the time, and leave to cool fully, stirring occasionally.

When cold, pour into an ice-cream machine and freeze following the manufacturer's instructions. Freeze until needed.

For the clafoutis, preheat the oven to 180°C/350°F/gas mark 4. Place all the ingredients except the raisins and the pineapple in a mixing bowl and, using a hand blender or whisk, beat to a smooth batter. Stir in the raisins and leave the batter to sit for 15 minutes.

Divide the pineapple cubes equally between 4 individual baking dishes, then pour over the sweet batter.

Bake for 25–30 minutes until golden. Allow to cool slightly. Top with a ball of curry ice cream and serve. If you're still not sure, vanilla ice cream works well, too!

4 PORTIONS: 497 KCALS, 17G PROTEIN, 16G FAT, 5.2G SATURATED FAT, 75G CARBOHYDRATE, 68.1G SUGAR, 1.6G FIBRE, 0.48G SALT, 189MG SODIUM

sweet fennel risotto

Fennel! In a dessert I hear you say! Don't knock it until you've tried it! Blanching the rice in the first stages of the recipe gives a less starchy grain and to me improves the final result. This is also delicious served cold, but I prefer it warm topped with fruits such as pears and apples. It makes a lovely warm and different dessert to serve on a cold winter night.

150g risotto rice (e.g. arborio, carnaroli)
20g unsalted butter (optional) or 1 tablespoon rapeseed oil
50g caster sugar
1 head fennel, trimmed and cut into small dice
100ml fresh or pre-packed pear juice
1 vanilla pod, halved and seeds removed
   (or 1 teaspoon vanilla extract)
600ml semi-skimmed milk, hot
50g raisins, soaked in water for 30 minutes until plump,
   drained and dried
½–1 pear, thinly sliced

Serves 4

Place the rice in a saucepan, cover it well with boiling water, simmer for 5 minutes, uncovered, then drain in a colander. Lightly rinse the rice under slow running water and set aside.

In a heavy-based pan, heat the butter and 20g of the sugar. When melted, add the fennel and cook over a low heat for 10–12 minutes until the fennel is tender and lightly caramelised.

Add the pear juice, remaining sugar, vanilla seeds and pods and bring to the boil. Add the hot milk and the blanched rice, reduce the heat and simmer for a further 20 minutes, stirring regularly, until the rice is cooked, creamy and still retaining a little bite to it.

Stir in the soaked raisins, then divide between 4 serving bowls. Drape thinly sliced raw pear over the risotto and serve.

4 PORTIONS: 326 KCALS, 9G PROTEIN, 6G FAT, 1.8G SATURATED FAT, 64G CARBOHYDRATE, 34.5G SUGAR, 2.2G FIBRE, 0.21G SALT, 81MG SODIUM

syrian winter fruits with saffron yogurt

To me dried fruits are very under-utilised, which is a shame, particularly as most (though not prunes) are high in potassium, which has the opposite effect in the body to sodium and helps reduce blood pressure! Here they are served warm with an aromatically flavoured saffron yogurt spiked with green cardamom. Dried limes are available from Middle Eastern stores, wonderful in many dishes of Arabic origin.

300ml orange juice
juice and zest of 1 lemon
1 cinnammon stick
½ teaspoon root ginger, chopped
2 tablespoons honey
1 dried lime, halved (optional)
400g ready-to-eat dried fruit
   (e.g. prunes, apricots, figs)

For the saffron yogurt
125ml low fat natural yogurt
1 teaspoon cornflour
½ teaspoon ground cardamom
good pinch of saffron (fresh
   or powder)

Serves 4

First heat the yogurt, saffron and cornflour together in a pan until it reaches the boil, stirring constantly. Cook for 1 minute, add the cardamom and remove to a bowl. Cool, then refrigerate for up to 2 hours.

For the fruit place the orange juice, lemon juice and zest, cinnamon, ginger, honey and dried lime in a pan. Bring to the boil then simmer for 5 minutes. Add the dried fruit, return to the boil, remove from the heat and leave to cool. Remove the fruit from the liquid then strain the poaching liquid. Return the poaching liquid to the pan and reduce it over a medium heat to syrup consistency.

To serve, warm the fruit gently in the syrup and divide between 4 serving dishes. Place a dollop of saffron yogurt to one side and serve.

4 PORTIONS: 242 KCALS, 5G PROTEIN, 1G FAT, 0.2G SATURATED FAT, 56G CARBOHYDRATE, 54.4G SUGAR, 6.4G FIBRE, 0.14G SALT, 56MG SODIUM

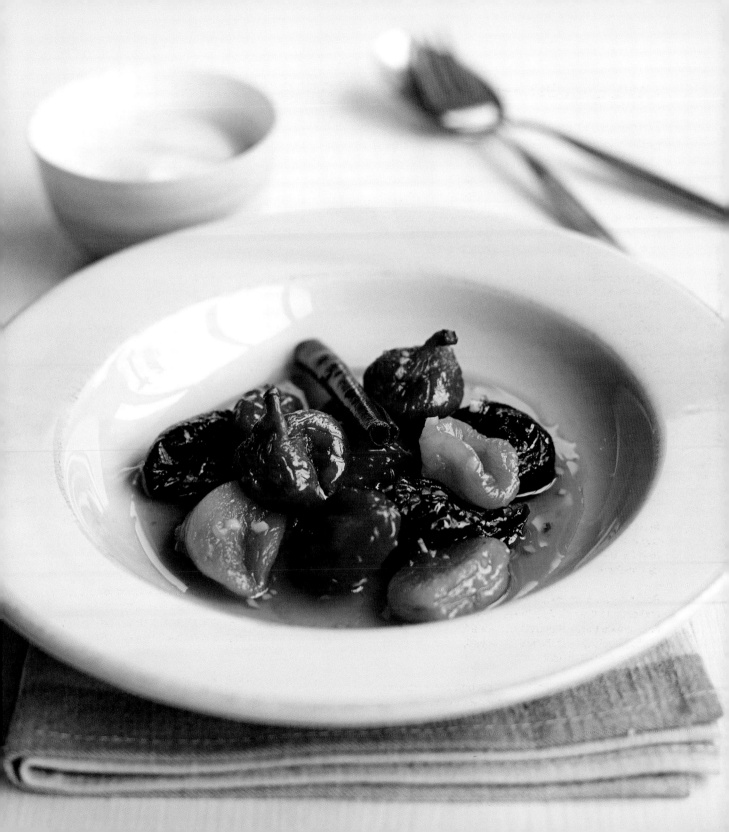

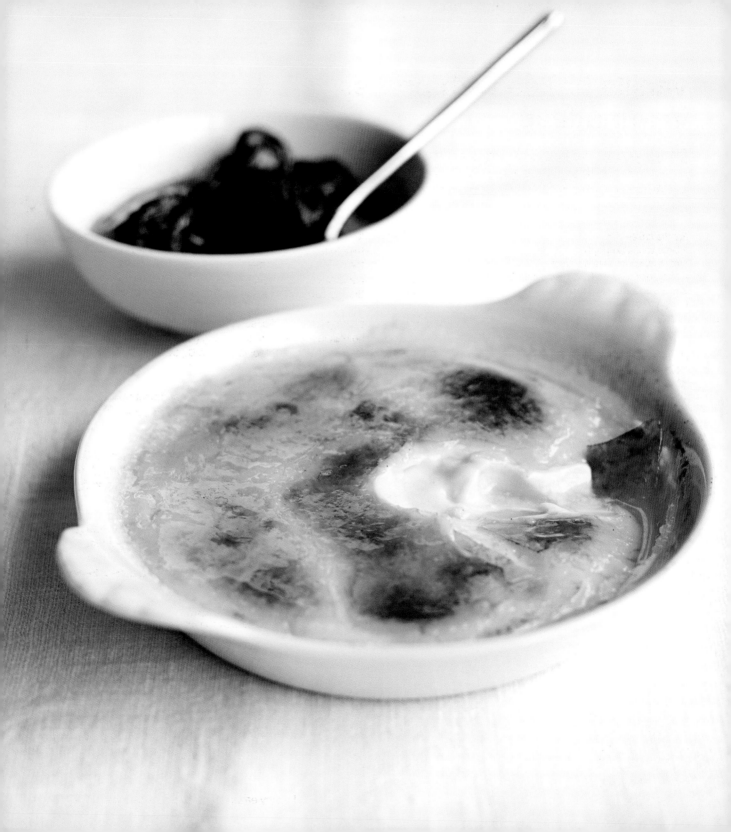

vanilla brûlée with prunes in armagnac

Everyone loves crème brûlée, traditionally made rich with double cream. My healthier version uses only milk, but with the vanilla and the Armagnac prunes is still packed with flavour. The prunes are best made well in advance.

For the brûlée
1 large vanilla pod, split
   (or 1 teaspoon vanilla extract)
600ml semi-skimmed milk, plus 2 tablespoons
2 tablespoons custard powder
6 egg yolks
70g caster sugar
1 tablespoon extra sugar, to glaze the brûlée

For the prunes
2 tablespoons maple syrup
12 large prunes, stoned and ready to eat
1 tablespoon Armagnac

Serves 4

For the prunes, bring the maple syrup and 100ml water to the boil and simmer for 5 minutes. Add the prunes and simmer for 5 minutes, then remove from the heat, add the Armagnac and allow to cool. Keep in a sealed container in the fridge. Note: the longer the prunes are left in the syrup, the better the flavour. They will keep well for up to a week.

For the brûlée, using a small knife, scrape the seeds from the vanilla pod, add to the milk in a small pan, then bring gently to the boil. Mix the custard powder with the extra 2 tablespoons milk, then whisk into the warm milk. Remove from the heat.

In a bowl, whisk together the egg yolks and sugar and beat until light and fluffy. Slowly whisk the thickened custard into the egg and whisk until smooth and creamy.

Return the custard to a low heat and cook until the custard is at 78°C (do not let it boil or curdle). Remove from the heat then strain through a fine sieve. Cool slightly. Pour into 4 gratin-style dishes, place in the fridge for 2–3 hours to set.

To serve, remove from the fridge, sprinkle liberally with sugar and, using a kitchen blow torch or under a preheated hot grill, glaze until golden.

Leave to cool about 2 minutes until the sugar crust has hardened. Serve with the Armagnac prunes on the side.

4 PORTIONS: 373 KCALS, 12G PROTEIN, 13G FAT, 4.4G SATURATED FAT, 54G CARBOHYDRATE, 48.6G SUGAR, 2.1G FIBRE, 0.27G SALT, 107MG SODIUM

stuffed baked apples with vanilla-cardamom yogurt

When I was young, baked apples were a regular option for dessert. Nowadays with all the various fruits we have available to buy and at our disposal, they have fallen from favour.

4 russet or golden delicious
  apples, stalks removed
75g dates, coarsely chopped
2 tablespoons flaked almonds
2 tablespoons shelled
  pistachio nuts
1 tablespoon brown sugar
juice of ½ lemon

For the vanilla-cardamom yogurt
125ml low-fat natural yogurt
1 vanilla pod, halved, seeds
  removed (or 1 teaspoon
  vanilla extract)
½ teaspoon ground cardamom
1 tablespoon maple syrup
pinch of ground cinnamon

Serves 4

Preheat the oven to 180°C/350°F/gas mark 4.

Core the apples with an apple corer, ensuring there are no pips or centre core remaining. You should have a clean, clear hollow through the middle from top to bottom.

In a bowl, mix together the remaining ingredients, then fill the centre of each apple with this mixture, pressing down to ensure the centre of each apple is fully filled. Place on a lightly greased baking tray.

Spoon 1 tablespoon hot water over each apple, then bake for 30–35 minutes until the apples are tender.

Meanwhile, combine all the ingredients for the vanilla-cardamom yogurt together in a bowl. Chill until needed.

Serve the stuffed apples warm with the yogurt sauce spooned over them.

4 PORTIONS: 447 KCALS, 8G PROTEIN, 18G FAT, 2.6G SATURATED FAT, 67G CARBOHYDRATE, 46.7G SUGAR, 9.8G FIBRE, 0.31G SALT, 122MG SODIUM

oriental style oranges with almond praline

When the blood orange season begins I often use them to prepare this dish, as their colour is so dramatic.

4 juicy medium-large oranges
50ml maple syrup
1 stick lemongrass, outer husk
  removed, remainder finely
  chopped
½ teaspoon chopped red chilli
2 star anise pods
4 passion fruits, halved, juice
  and seeds separated

1 small piece stem ginger,
  finely chopped, plus 1
  teaspoon syrup from the jar

For the praline
150g caster sugar
60g slivered almonds
seeds from passion fruits
  (see above)

Serves 4

For the praline, place the sugar and 45ml water in a small heavy-based pan and cook over a low heat until the sugar has dissolved. Without stirring, bring to the boil until the sugar caramelises and becomes golden amber in colour. Remove from the heat, stir in the almonds and passion fruit seeds, then pour into a small baking tray lined with greaseproof paper and leave to go hard. Break into large pieces and set aside.

For the oranges, thinly pare the zest from one orange then remove the peel from all the oranges and cut into thick slices.

Place the maple syrup, lemongrass, chilli, star anise, orange zest and 150ml water in a pan and simmer for 5 minutes. Remove from the heat and add the passion fruit juice and chopped ginger and syrup.

Arrange the orange slices on a deep plate, stacked on top of each other, pour over the syrup and chill until ready to serve. Top the oranges with the almond praline and serve chilled.

4 PORTIONS: 303 KCALS, 4G PROTEIN, 9G FAT, 0.6G SATURATED FAT, 56G CARBOHYDRATE, 54.4G SUGAR, 2.3G FIBRE, 0.33G SALT, 11MG SODIUM

wild berry cranachan

Made with low-fat yogurt instead of the usual cream, this traditional Scottish dessert is often served at a New Year or Burns' Night festivities. Originally known as 'cream crowdie' as the dessert was made using crowdie, a curd cheese that is soft and crumbly with a slightly sour taste. Use vanilla extract rather than essence for the dish: there is a great vanilla extract from Nielsen Massey available in most good supermarkets, look out for it.

100g porridge oats
275ml low-fat natural yogurt
1 tablespoon reduced-sugar raspberry jam
1 teaspoon vanilla extract
1 tablespoon honey
1 tablespoon whisky

300g mixed wild berries of your choice (e.g. blueberries, blackberries, raspberries, loganberries)

Serves 4

Place the oats in a hot, dry non-stick frying pan, and heat for about 1 minute until lightly golden (alternatively, spread the oats out on a baking tray and place under a hot grill).

In a bowl, mix the yogurt, jam, vanilla, honey and whisky. Crush 225g of the fruit lightly in a bowl, then gently fold in the yogurt mix. Finally fold through the toasted oats, leaving a few to garnish the top, using a metal spoon to give a rippled effect.

Transfer to tall glasses, top with the remaining berries, sprinkle over the remaining toasted oats and serve.

4 PORTIONS: 180 KCALS, 8G PROTEIN, 3G FAT, 0.7G SATURATED FAT, 31G CARBOHYDRATE, 14G SUGAR, 4.5G FIBRE, 0.12G SALT, 48MG SODIUM

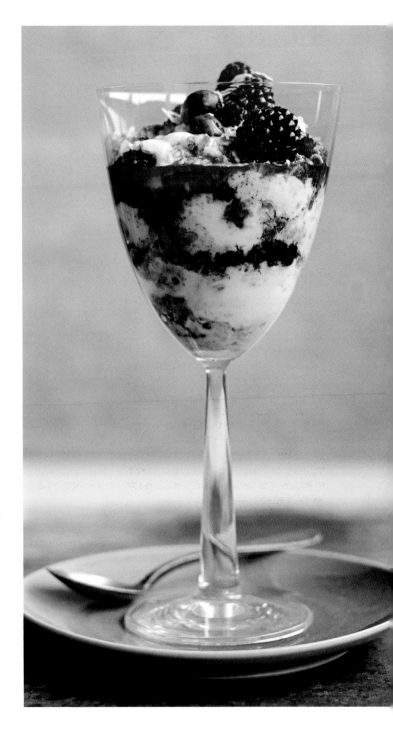

stock bases

You will notice that I use a lot of freshly made stocks in my recipes. The reason for this is two fold:

Firstly, commercial stock cubes are rather salty in flavour, thereby defeating the object of reducing your salt intake and secondly, homemade stocks not only taste better but give a much better flavour to the dish you are cooking.

There are some fairly acceptable ambient stocks available in sachet form from leading supermarkets and delis but make sure you look out for the reduced-salt varieties. If you are intent on using a stock cube, I recommend using only half a cube per 600ml of liquid.

Homemade stocks take very little time and effort to make and can be prepared in advance, kept covered in the fridge for up to 4 days or in the freezer for up to 3 months, in small quantities.

chicken stock

2 kg chicken bones
2 medium onions, chopped
2 sticks celery, chopped
1 bay leaf
2 medium carrots, chopped
2 teaspoons black peppercorns
5 litres water

Combine all the ingredients in a large pan, bring to the boil and skim off any impurities which rise to the surface. Simmer for 2 hours, then strain (makes 2.5 litres).

reduced chicken stock

As for the chicken stock but first roast all the dry ingredients in the oven for 30 minutes with 1 tablespoon tomato purée until golden. Drain off any excess fat, then place in a pan and simmer for 2 hours, then strain.

Place in a pan, bring to the boil and simmer until the liquid has reduced by half (makes 1.5 litres). This will give a darker, more complex flavour that is often used in sauce bases.

fish stock

1.5 kg fish bones
1 medium onion, chopped
2 stick celery, chopped
1 bay leaf
½ teaspoon black peppercorns
4 litres water

Combine all the ingredients in a large pan and bring to the boil. Simmer uncovered for 20 minutes, skimming off the impurities that rise to the surface, then strain (makes 2.5 litres).

vegetable stock

1 large carrot, chopped
1 large parsnip, chopped
2 medium onions, chopped
2 carrots, chopped
2 sticks celery, chopped
1 bay leaf
1 teaspoon black peppercorns
4 litres water

Combine all the ingredients in a large pan, bring to the boil, simmer uncovered for 1 hour, then strain (makes 2.5 litres).

index

acknowledgements

Working on this book has not only been an enjoyable culinary challenge but also extremely educational for me and having the support of Gemma Heiser has benefited the book no end. Thank you Gemma for all your knowledge and support.

As always, my heartfelt thanks go to home economist and friend Linda Tubby and photographer Will Heap. Thank you both for your boundless enthusiasm, passion and dedication to this project.

Thanks also to Wendy Doyle for analysing the recipes from a nutritional standpoint, Roisin Nield for her beautiful prop styling, Geoff Hayes, for his stunning book design, and Gemma John, for taking care of the production side of things.

Many thanks to Lara Mand, my PA, for her help in formulating the backbone of the recipes in the early stages.

And finally, a huge thank you to Judith Hannam, editor, and Vicki Murrell, editorial assistant, for their invaluable support and friendship. Working with you both has been effortless and a real pleasure. You helped see the project through every stage and I am very grateful to you both for making it all happen.

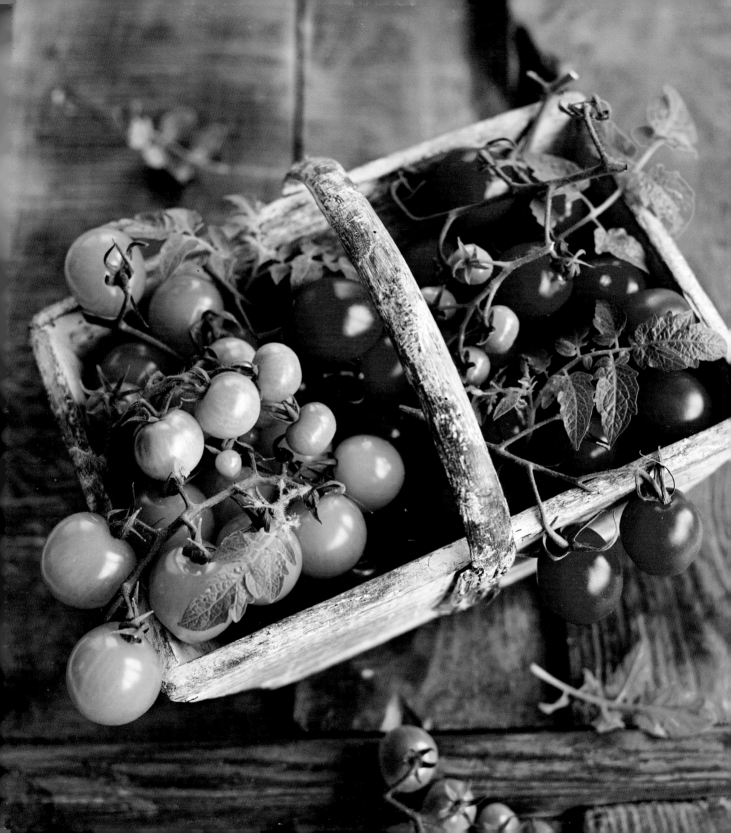